A TIME TO BE BORN
AND A TIME TO DIE

Starkoff Institute Studies
in Ethics and
Contemporary Moral Problems

A TIME TO BE BORN AND A TIME TO DIE

The Ethics of Choice

Barry S. Kogan

Editor

ALDINE DE GRUYTER

New York

About the Editor

Barry S. Kogan is Professor of Jewish Philosophy at Hebrew Union College-Jewish Institute of Religion, Cincinnati, Ohio and Director of The Starkoff Institute of Ethics and Contemporary Moral Problems. He is the author of *Averroes and the Metaphysics of Causation* and editor of *Spinoza: A Tercentenary Perspective.*

ALDINE DE GRUYTER
A division of Walter de Gruyter, Inc.
200 Saw Mill River Road
Hawthorne, New York 10532

The paper used in this publication meets the minimum requirements of American National Standard for Information Sciences—Permanence of Paper for Printed Library Materials, ANSI Z39.48-1984. ⊚

Library of Congress Cataloging-in-Publication Data
A Time to be born and a time to die : the ethics of choice / edited by
  Barry S. Kogan.
      p.   cm.
    Revised versions of papers presented at a conference, held on Oct. 15–17, 1989 in Cincinnati, Ohio, sponsored by the Hebrew Union College-Jewish Institute of Religion through its Starkoff Institute of Ethics and Contemporary Moral Problems.
    Includes bibliographical references and index.
    ISBN 0-202-30388-8 (cloth : alk. paper). — ISBN 0-202-30389-6
(paper :alk. paper)
    1. Medical ethics—Congresses. I. Kogan, Barry S. II. Hebrew Union College-Jewish Institute of Religion. III. Starkoff Institute of Ethics and Contemporary Moral Problems.
    [DNLM: 1. Ethics, Medical—congresses. 2. Religion and Medicine—congresses. 3. Right to Die—congresses. 4. Technology, Medical—congresses. W 50 T583]
R724.T55   1991
174'.2—dc20
DNLM/DLC
for Library of Congress   91-6504
                                                                              CIP

Manufactured in the United States of America

10 9 8 7 6 5 4 3 2 1

To Steffi

רַבּוֹת בָּנוֹת עָשׂוּ חָיִל וְאַתְּ עָלִית עַל כֻּלָּנָה

"Many women have done well,
But you surpass them all."

Proverbs 31:29

Contents

Acknowledgments

Although a book often has only one author or editor, it is invariably the work of many devoted hands. I am happy for the opportunity to record here my sincere thanks to all of those who have contributed their best efforts to bringing this volume to completion. It was through the generosity of Bernard J. and Florence Starkoff and the initiative and encouragement of Alfred Gottschalk, President of Hebrew Union College-Jewish Institute of Religion, that the Starkoff Institute of Ethics was created and its commitment to meaningful education on contemporary moral problems established. They, together with David H. Ellenson, John J. Raymond, Jr., Jerome S. Rubin, and Henry R. Winkler, all members of the Institute board, played a major role in determining the theme and structure of the conference that generated this volume.

Josef E. Fischer, Chairman of the Department of Surgery at the University of Cincinnati College of Medicine, and Kenneth Ehrlich, Dean of the Cincinnati campus of HUC-JIR, are to be thanked for smoothing the path that led to this volume in many ways and for offering much good counsel in the process. Ida Rubin was particularly helpful in arranging for the graphic design used on the cover of this volume, and I would like to express my sincere appreciation for her efforts. I also want to thank Marion Magid, managing editor of *Commentary* magazine, for permission to reprint those excerpts of Leon Kass' article, "Death with Dignity and the Sanctity of Life," which appeared in the March 1990 issue of *Commentary.* I am particularly grateful to Richard Koffler of Aldine de Gruyter for his consistent support of this project and for his helpful suggestions during the editorial process.

Good friends and colleagues have offered many valuable editorial suggestions at various stages in preparing the manuscript. I would like to express my deep appreciation to Pat Gibbons, Michael Meyer, Lynn Sommers, Judy Feintuch, and Leon Kass for their perceptive comments. I also want to thank Deborah Diamond, who joined our staff on various special occasions and whose resourcefulness and dedication always helped us to get the job done.

To my administrative assistant, Phyllis Binik-Thomas, I owe a special debt of thanks. Her many talents, winning manner, and ability to work so very well under all kinds of circumstances have helped to make the editing process as enjoyable as it was rewarding.

Finally, words alone cannot adequately express the gratitude I feel to my wife, Steffi. Through her love and encouragement, she has made all of the tasks connected with producing this volume easier to achieve and all the more worth doing. Together with my children, Avi and Elana, she has made the most important things possible. To her this volume is joyfully dedicated.

Introduction

Barry S. Kogan

"A season is set for everything, a time for every experience under heaven: A time for being born and a time for dying, a time for planting and a time for uprooting what is planted" (*Eccl.* 3:1–2). In measured cadences that evoke the pre-determined order he sets out to describe, the author of *Ecclesiastes* focuses our attention on what today we would call "the facts of life" or "the way things really are." He tells us that life has limits that are not of our making and that are largely beyond our ken. What unfolds between birth and death is an unpredictable succession of opposing activities and events allotted to us by an inscrutable God. We may strive to discover what we can about future events—either to profit from their occurrence or to avoid the pain they might bring—but ultimately we shall strive in vain. The wisest course is to face these facts and renounce our ceaseless striving after what we cannot know and cannot have, at least without sacrificing the real good of human life that we can achieve and also enjoy (*Eccl.* 3:12). As one recent commentator sums up this teaching, "The fruit of wisdom is not the accumulation of all knowledge and the understanding of all mysteries. It lies rather in recognizing the limitations of human knowledge and power. Man is not the measure of all things. He is the master neither of life nor of death. He can find serenity only in coming to terms with the unalterable conditions of his existence and enjoying its real but limited satisfactions."[1] Whether this vision was elaborated in pietistic or philosophic terms during subsequent generations, its commitment to a wise and principled acceptance of life's limits has long played an important role in the development of our moral traditions.

Yet it is by now a familiar story that in the sixteenth and seventeenth centuries a very different attitude and response to the "unalterable conditions" of human existence arose. Proponents of the new empirical

1

science committed themselves, as never before, to the study of nature and its conditions. They readily conceded that the ultimate character of things still remained unknown and perhaps unknowable as well. But they argued confidently that the *observed* workings of nature could nevertheless become the basis of a new natural science, far more precise and secure in its findings than anything attained by the ancients or the medievals. The goal of their observations and inquiries would be knowledge as before, but it would not be simply knowledge pursued for its own sake or to actualize our understanding. Rather it would be knowledge understood as power over nature, that is, power to alter as far as possible the unalterable conditions of human existence "for the relief of man's estate."[2]

Writing in 1665, Robert Hooke, the English experimental philosopher and curator to the Royal Society, captured well the remarkable optimism that accompanied this bold scientific project. At the same time, however, he pointed—perhaps unintentionally—to the moral ambiguity which accompanied it as well.

> If once this method were followed with diligence and attention, there is nothing that lies within the power of human wit (or which is far more effectual) of human industry, which we might not encompass; we might not only hope for inventions to equal those of Copernicus, Galileo, Gilbert, Harvey, and of others, whose names are almost lost, that were the inventors of gun-powder, the seaman's compass, printing, etching, graving, microscopes, etc. but multitudes that may far exceed them. For even those discoveries seem to have been the products of some such method, though but imperfect. What may not be therefore expected from it if thoroughly prosecuted? Talking and contention of arguments would soon be turned into labors; all the fine dreams of opinions and universal metaphysical natures, which the luxury of subtle brains have devised, would quickly vanish and give place to solid histories, experiments, and works. And as at first, mankind fell by tasting of the forbidden Tree of Knowledge, so we, their posterity, may be in part restored by the same way, not only by beholding and contemplating, but by tasting too those fruits of natural knowledge, that were never yet forbidden. From hence the world may be assisted with [a] variety of inventions, new matter for the sciences collected, [and] the old improved . . . .[3]

The possibilities for discovery seemed truly limitless, but it was not discovery alone that stirred these new experimental philosophers. The attraction was ultimately more practical than it was intellectual. It was the prospect of harnessing the powers of human reason to human industry in order to assist the world by producing all kinds of inventions. The reward for creating a scientific technology capable of altering the natural conditions of human life would be at least a partial "restoration" to the more congenial conditions we associate with the story of Eden.

Compared to such a project, ancient and medieval arguments about the true nature of things seemed fruitless. Mere opinions about the good life for human beings would have to give way to the activity of creating it.

Still, there was a moral ambiguity implicit in this early scientific utopianism that even its ardent supporters like Hooke recognized. The restoration they contemplated was to be achieved *in the same way* that mankind originally fell—"by tasting of the forbidden Tree of Knowledge." In other words, relief of man's estate, like the "fall" into it, would come about through autonomous action by human beings rejecting in some way the divine or natural constraints that had always been part of human life. It would come also by "tasting the fruits of natural knowledge that were never yet forbidden," in effect, by enjoying the results of the technology that were now identified with the Tree of Life. But this is where the moral difficulty lies. Can human welfare and flourishing be attained by using some means that are forbidden along with others that are not? Are the technological fruits of natural knowledge unambiguously life-giving, as if they had fallen from the Tree of Life? Or are they not more like a mixed blessing akin to the presumably hybrid fruit of the Tree of Knowledge of Good *and* Evil? Can we, in sum, hope to relieve man's estate without reflecting continually on what relief is and what we gain and lose in trying to attain it?[4]

Hooke and his colleagues, of course, did not raise these questions and would probably have considered them essentially scholastic and theoretical. It would only be many generations later, when the fruits of scientific technology became available in abundance, that they would come to the forefront of inquiry as matters of intensely practical concern. That time has surely arrived, and general concern with such questions has never been more practical or intense than it is now in the realm of medicine and health.

Perhaps more than any other field, modern medicine has been seen as the embodiment of the humane aspirations and high hopes of the scientific revolution. Its twin aims of promoting health and curing disease made it the natural candidate to change the conditions of human life for the better. Its foundation in experience and experiment as well as its receptivity to technological innovation made it a ready example of what scientific progress could really achieve. Clearly, medicine's greatest achievement has been its growing capacity to control the conditions of life and of death. From the conquest of infectious diseases to the repair of accidental injuries to the campaign against degenerative disease, breakthroughs have come in increasingly rapid succession. In our own generation, the development of oral contraceptives, fertility drugs, *in vitro* fertilization, embryo transfer, amniocentesis, sonograms, surgical correction of fetal abnormalities, and the technology both to maintain fetal viability outside the womb and to conduct medically safe abortions has revolutionized the circumstances under which life begins as well as our understanding of that beginning. Similarly, the development of life-prolonging interventions such as kidney dialysis, cardiac pacemakers, open-heart surgery, organ transplantation, ventilators, cardio-pulmonary resuscitation, angioplasty, the artificial heart, and the life-support technology of the modern intensive care unit has radically altered the circumstances under which death occurs and even our definition of death itself. Few, indeed, are those who have not been touched in some way by these advances.

The rapid pace of technological change in medicine in the past several decades has inevitably generated both serious interest and intense controversy over the social and moral implications of these developments. This is only natural. As Daniel Callahan has observed, "rapid technologic change forces a confrontation with received values and moral principles. The moral vision that gave coherence and guidance in the past under one set of social conditions appears threatened by new and disruptive conditions. And what could be newer and more disruptive than biomedically induced changes in mankind's ancient struggle with illness and death?"[5] Thus, ethical dilemmas have arisen in virtually every area of biomedical research and health care delivery. Physicians and nurses alike have felt a growing need to re-examine and reformulate standards of professional conduct. Hospital administrators as well as medical, nursing, and support staff have sought new policy guidelines to deal with previously unforeseen situations for which they are often held morally and legally responsible. Patients have increasingly claimed the right to a greater say in their own treatment.

All of these factors have contributed significantly to the rise of biomedical ethics as a distinct professional field. Drawing on the resources of medicine, biology, law, religion, philosophy, and the social sciences, it has produced a burgeoning professional literature in response to all these needs. It has established institutions for the training of bioethicists holding advanced degrees to serve in hospitals, medical schools, universities, research centers, institutional review boards, and government commissions in the United States and many other nations. Most important, it has strived to educate health care professionals and the general public alike about the moral problems and possibilities that accompany our quest for better health.

The essays that follow are an attempt to advance that practical, educational goal. They represent original studies by many of the leading figures in biomedical ethics today. Their names and works are already well known both inside and outside the field. What they have written here significantly expands and updates their previously published work on the topics addressed and thus represents their latest thinking about these issues. In addition, the volume has been deliberately arranged to allow for significant dialogue and interchange between the contributors wherever possible. In this way, alternative views of the same moral dilemmas and appraisals of arguments offered to resolve them stand out as the live options that their proponents maintain they are and in ways that encourage readers to think through the issues and decide for themselves.

Earlier versions of all these essays were presented at a major conference on bioethics, also entitled "A Time to be Born and a Time to Die: The Ethics of Choice," held on October 15–17, 1989 in Cincinnati, Ohio. The conference was sponsored by the Hebrew Union College-Jewish Institute of Religion through its Starkoff Institute of Ethics and Contemporary Moral Problems. The goal of the program was to provide a forum for concerned health care professionals, bioethicists, academicians, and clergy to gain a better understanding of the impact of current medical and technological advances on the ethics of prenatal and neonatal care as well as the medical treatment of the aging and the terminally ill. As the oldest rabbinical seminary in North America, the College-Institute has long had an intense interest in the application of our received moral traditions to the changing realities of modern life. In pursuing that interest, it established the Starkoff Institute of Ethics to bring together distinguished leaders from various fields in order to identify emerging sources of moral conflict, to explore the assumptions and value-frameworks that guide our decision making, and to develop educational materials from these meetings that can prepare future professionals to make informed and morally sound decisions in their life's work.

The title of the conference and of the volume was selected for several reasons. First, the citation from *Ecclesiastes* calls attention to the fact that while birth and death are seen as opposites, they are not for that reason unrelated. They are traditionally understood as the limiting occasions that begin and end a single human life. Accordingly, any coherent view of what it is to be a human being, to whom obligations are owed, must seriously consider when it is that a human life, however undeveloped, begins and when it is that the same life, however diminished, really ends. Second, life-prolonging technologies and other interventions have greatly altered both the times and circumstances of birth and death. Most of the controversies that have stirred public interest and concern with bioethics thus far center on the beginning and the end of life. It therefore becomes necessary to rethink the content of our obligations to other human beings in just these circumstances and to understand what principles have guided our thinking until now and what adjustments may be called for in the future. Third, the reference to

"The Ethics of Choice" was not meant to endorse either a particular philosophy or ideology of choice or the principle that choosing is the supreme ethical value. Rather, it is there to indicate that what is ultimately at stake in our choices is their ethical character. In short, we need to choose well.

This collection of essays is divided into three parts. The first, "Surveying Current Issues," takes up a number of bioethical problems that are currently receiving a great deal of public attention and discusses both their moral and legal ramifications in historical context. The second, "Rethinking Controversial Questions," is devoted to an in-depth analysis of either a single issue or a closely related complex of issues that has been a focus of intense debate from a variety of philosophic, religious, and public policy perspectives. The third and final part, "Drawing Guidance from Our Traditions," explores some methodological problems and possibilities for appropriating moral norms from the Jewish and Christian religious traditions and applying them meaningfully when we face mortal choices in the modern world.

Ruth Macklin opens Part I with a survey of mortal choices today as they affect the rights of patients to participate in decisions affecting their treatment. Noting that paternalism on the part of physicians toward their patients has been greatly reduced, she argues that the main impediments to recognition of patients' rights now come from other quarters, and she identifies various dilemmas of justice deriving from each one. Hospital administrators and risk managers tend to encourage overtreating patients out of fear of legal liability. In doing so, they disenfranchise them. Cost-containment efforts and competition for scarce resources leave other patients, especially poorer ones, undertreated and ignorant of the criteria by which medical resources are allocated. Patients who contribute to their own diseases through drug or alcohol abuse find themselves denied transplants and other benefits on largely arbitrary grounds. Diagnosis of maternal–fetal conflict situations, in turn, has led to increased efforts to coerce or control pregnant women on behalf of their unborn offspring. She proposes several criteria, consistent with recognition of patients' rights, to resolve these situations, while acknowledging that consensus will nonetheless be hard to achieve.

George Annas analyzes the history and legal ramifications of the right of privacy in American law in terms of decisions affecting the beginning of life, the end of life, and the links between both. After tracing the right of privacy to the concept of personal liberty expressed in the Fourteenth Amendment, he argues that current debates about privacy ultimately hinge on whether to use the criminal law to support only the morality of duty, which any society needs to survive, or also the morality of aspiration, which endorses a generally accepted vision of the good.

Through a detailed examination of cases such as *Roe* v. *Wade*, the *Webster* decision, the *Cruzan* case, and that of Angela Carder, among others, he contends that issues of birth and death properly belong to the morality of aspiration. Attempts to bring the criminal law to bear on cases involving abortion and the right to refuse treatment succeed only in making these extraordinarily difficult decisions seem simple and clear-cut. Conversely, they fail to take into account either the individual's personal beliefs, or the wishes of family members, or the personal dignity of those most affected. Thus, when there are strong moral disagreements between major segments of a society, Annas concludes that it is inappropriate and unwise to look to the criminal law for solutions.

Part II, "Rethinking Controversial Questions," begins with Daniel Callahan's probing discussion of how the debate about abortion has evolved over the past 30 years. He sees the continuing controversy as a case study in the problems and paradoxes of "the pluralistic proposition," especially for the pro-choice position, which he himself espouses as the only viable option for our society. The pluralistic proposition holds that the law should leave decisions about essentially private acts that lack a basic moral consensus and do not harm other people to individual conscience. The question that it raises is whether a strong notion of pluralism necessarily requires a weak notion of personal morality or whether, instead, it is possible to nourish a strong and meaningful sense of morality in a pluralistic society that nevertheless preserves choice. In analyzing and critically evaluating the arguments of both sides, but especially those used by the pro-choice movement both before and after *Roe* v. *Wade*, he finds that the latter has increasingly displayed a strong commitment to legal freedom and women's rights along with a weak commitment to substantive moral examination of choice. He argues that this is a narrow and unsatisfactory combination, which in the long run will be self-defeating as well. In its place he proposes a more nuanced position that recognizes the need for serious public debate about personal moral choices, accepts the necessity of compromises in the law, and acts to change the economic and social circumstances that lead women to make coerced choices for abortion. Such a position, he maintains, would better serve both the interests of the pro-choice movement and the pluralistic proposition itself.

Mark Washofsky responds to Callahan from the perspective of a liberal Jew likewise committed to the pro-choice position. He agrees on the need for building that position on strong moral foundations but finds the pluralistic proposition, by nature, inadequate to the task. Instead he proposes the example of the Jewish legal tradition, which is one of the principal sources of both our respect for life and our respect for human freedom, to serve as such a foundation. He shows that biblical and

rabbinic law neither treat the destruction of a fetus as murder nor warrant abortion as justified under all circumstances. Rather, the tradition
leaves the decision to competent rabbinic authorities acting on a case-by-
case basis in conjunction with those directly affected. It also acknowledges the legitimacy of principled disagreement within the same moral
tradition. Accordingly, Washofsky expresses concern that compromises
to restrict abortion in the post-*Webster* era may have the awkward result
of denying individuals the opportunity to make choices that are morally
justified within their own tradition. Compromises that are inevitably
political in character, he concludes, should not be confused with serious
moral debate.

In his role as both a genetic and pastoral counselor in the Methodist
tradition, Frank Seydel explores a variety of moral dilemmas that arise
from the use of organs from anencephalic donors, fetal tissue research,
and counseling individuals and families about genetic defects. Controversy over using organs from anencephalic infants centers on questions
surrounding their status as living persons and when it is permissible to
use their organs for transplantation. After examining current practices
and positions on these issues, he defends an emerging consensus that
such infants should be accorded at least the minimum respect that we
accord other members of the species. The main dilemma in fetal research
is the status of the fetus and controversy about the means of acquiring
fetal tissue, namely, abortion. Since both issues are not likely to be
resolved until the abortion controversy is itself resolved, Seydel endorses a compromise proposed by Kathleen Nolan that only fetal tissue
from aborted ectopic pregnancies (in which both the mother and the
fetus will die without the abortion) should be used for research. Finally,
he identifies three major challenges now faced by genetic counselors—
abortion, the detection of nonpaternity, and confidentiality—and discusses various ways in which counselors can help families to cope effectively with the often tragic results of genetic screening.

Fred Rosner addresses these and other issues as a practicing physician
committed to traditional Jewish law. Its central teaching is that human
life is a divine gift of infinite value, which human beings are obliged to
preserve. In the light of recent developments in fetal therapy and surgery, he discusses a growing tendency to differentiate the fetus from the
mother for therapeutic purposes and the maternal–fetal conflict situations that often result from it. In general, he contends that if the risk to
the mother is small, she is obliged to let the fetus be treated for correctable conditions. But if the risk is great, she has no such obligation because
her life takes precedence. After exploring in detail reasons for and
against using organs from anencephalic infants, he argues for developing ways to care for them while they show signs of independent respira-

tion. Once respiration ceases or brain death is verified, there is no objection to using their organs to save other lives. Finally, he discusses genetic screening and counseling based on his experience with Tay-Sachs disease. Noting that even a handicapped fetus has a right to be born, other things being equal, he nevertheless gives qualified endorsement to screening and counseling programs, if strict confidentiality is guaranteed and sensitivity to both the religious commitment and the health needs of clients is shown.

Leon Kass explores what is meant in human terms by notions such as the sanctity of life, human dignity, and death with dignity, especially when the latter is increasingly identified with various forms of euthanasia and assisted suicide. He argues first that using the language of rights and duties in situations when human beings face death is poorly suited to determining what the best course of action is. Such language shifts our focus from doing what is right to fulfilling escalating demands that have both contradictory and mischievous results. He maintains that, contrary to prevailing assumptions, the sanctity of life and death with dignity are not only compatible with one another, but actually go hand in hand once they are properly understood. The reason is that the parallel notions of the sanctity and dignity of human life are grounded neither in the individual will nor in the conventional agreement of society, but in the very being of man as intrinsically god-like and essentially characterized by the attributes of speech, reason, freedom, judgment, and care. While disease and excessive medical treatment may undermine human dignity, they do not insult or deny it as taking life would. Death with dignity, therefore, has more to do with exercising at all times the human virtues that make life possible than with medical procedures that might cause death. He concludes by arguing that active euthanasia and assisted suicide will not promote either human dignity or the kind of death that affirms it, but rather will subvert both dignified conduct and decency in human relationships.

After noting a number of concerns he shares with Kass about the care of the terminally ill and euthanasia, Ronald Green goes on to discuss several points of disagreement over "moral methodology" and its practical implications. In terms of theory, he maintains that Kass's account of the sanctity of life sets up a false dichotomy between either respecting life because the individual or society wills it so or respecting life because it is intrinsically worthy of respect. The dichotomy overlooks a third alternative, namely, that rational persons pursuing various aims might nonetheless choose to limit the sovereignty of their wills for rational ends. This view, he suggests, better explains both our prohibitions of consensual killing and coercion and exceptions to the sanctity principle than does Kass's appeal to self-evident intuitions and religious arguments. In practical terms, Green points out that making rational willing the basis for our moral norms does not imply that every expression of a person's will must be respected, especially when he or she consents to active euthanasia. But it does allow for a more nuanced consideration of when it is rational to want to die, even with assistance, and when it is not, in comparison with Kass's basic rejection of this wish. Thus, he concludes that dignity has many meanings, and one of them involves having some control over the circumstances of one's life and death.

As a member of the National Institutes of Health Data Safety and Monitoring Board, LeRoy Walters discusses several important moral questions about research and public policy in his account of the randomized clinical trials that led to the approval of AZT in treating persons with AIDS or HIV infection. He describes the history of two research protocols designed to test the efficacy, toxicity, and recommended dosage of the new drug for high-risk patients with early symptoms of AIDS and for asymptomatic patients who tested positive for HIV. The practical issues that the monitoring board faced included such problems as what balance of therapeutic efficacy against toxicity constituted an acceptable risk, when to regard clear but incomplete test results as sufficient to stop the trial, and what to do about parallel clinical trials then ongoing. Walters describes the board's actions and deliberations on these issues and then examines the implications of the trial's principal finding that it is critical for people at risk for HIV infection to be tested and treated. He shows that (1) in the current social context it is rational both for at-risk individuals to decide to be tested and to forego being tested, and (2) there is as yet no evidence that knowledge of antibody status has resulted in safer sex. He concludes by outlining the main elements of an ethically acceptable public policy to deal with the HIV epidemic and by identifying some unresolved problems that might attend it. With other members of the monitoring board, he sees the epidemic not only as a tragedy, but also as an opportunity to address the larger problem of equal access to health care in our society.

Expressing fundamental agreement with Leroy Walters' conclusions based on similar IRB experience of her own, Carol Levine describes the historical context of human subjects research in the United States and examines several of the policy implications that follow from Walters' discussion. She notes that the FDA's current lifting of regulatory barriers on largely untested drugs follows a long period of establishing protection against scandal and abuse in such research. One benefit of this change is the attempt to include previously underrepresented groups such as pregnant women, children, and minority group members—all hard hit by AIDS—in such tests; but problems of access continue to undermine the change in policy. Other difficulties arise in testing for and treating asymptomatic HIV-infected infants because there is currently no way to determine whether testing positive indicates genuine infection in the baby or in the mother only. Levine then offers an independent analysis of the risks and benefits of "early intervention" once HIV infection has been reliably diagnosed. She concludes her essay with a discussion of the reasons for and against mandatory screening of adults and children and argues strongly against both for a variety of moral reasons. However, once improved therapies exist, she notes that there will be a need for both dramatically expanded services to treat those who have tested positive and increased efforts to protect the right of individuals to privacy and confidentiality.

James Childress analyzes the problem of fairness in allocating health care by examining the case of organ transplantation as a realistic index of the ethical, social, medical, and scientific factors at work in making appropriate choices. Proceeding from the principle that donated organs are scarce public resources to be used for the welfare of the community, he discusses in detail such issues as standards of justice in distributing donated organs, criteria for establishing waiting lists and for selecting organ recipients, evaluating point systems, the appropriateness of the "ability to pay" as a criterion of access, and questions of priority in funding and support. He defines justice as "rendering each person his or her due" and argues that selection must not be based on morally irrelevant characteristics like race or sex. A combination of medically verifiable need and the probability of a successful outcome (medical utility) represents for Childress the fairest criterion for establishing a waiting list. Although he acknowledges that women, minority groups, and low-income patients have disproportionately low representation on waiting lists and allows that affirmative action may be necessary to correct such inequities, he nonetheless maintains that fairness to donors requires the efficient use of donated organs. He goes on to offer a sympathetic analysis of the arguments of the federal Task Force on Organ Transplantation for increased funding and then to discuss the problem of macroallocation of health care resources, that is, determining which technologies, which diseases, and what kind of health care (prevention, chronic, or critical care) should receive which resources. He concludes that when there are conflicts between fundamental moral principles, it is not possible to know in advance which one should be given priority. Because the context of such conflicts is always changing, the search for balance over time requires constant clarification of the issues and continual readjustment.

In his response, Robert Veatch acknowledges that justice is only one of several principles that could make a policy right. He goes on to argue that justice should be construed primarily as giving people the opportunity for equality of well-being. By this standard, strictly speaking, justice would not require using scarce resources to benefit the least well-off, or individuals who choose risky life styles, or those with a lower health status, although other principles very well might do so. In terms of allocating organs, Veatch strongly criticizes Childress' identification of patient need and the probability of a successful transplant as medical utility. He also rejects treating medical utility as a principle of fairness because appeals to medical utility actually suspend the principle of equal concern and respect for those in need. Only luck determines who will actually have the best outcome. Again, tissue matching is not truly random because we know that members of disadvantaged minority groups are difficult to match. In examining age as a criterion for matching, Veatch also rejects Daniel Callahan's conception of a natural life span and proposes the "over a lifetime perspective" as the basis for claims to equal opportunity for well-being. Finally, he criticizes the strategy of balancing the competing claims of justice and medical effectiveness in decisions about macroallocation because such attempts at balance further dilute the commitment to equality of well-being and raise the dangerous prospect of sacrificing individuals against their will to some aggregate social good.

The third and final part of the book, "Drawing Guidance from our Traditions," opens with David Ellenson's discussion of two influential models for eliciting guidance from the Jewish tradition on contemporary biomedical issues. He holds that methodology plays a crucial role in determining what kind of guidance is derived from the sources, what form it takes, and who is judged competent to provide it. The first method, which he characterizes as *"halakhic* formalism," draws mainly on the Jewish legal tradition of *halakhah* by identifying precedents in the literature, inferring practical norms from them, and then reasoning by analogy to contemporary applications. Using debates about brain death and euthanasia as illustrations, he shows how this approach accommodates a plurality of norms within the system and yet places constraints on individual autonomy. The second or "covenantal" approach finds the case-law tradition too narrow to deal effectively with contemporary realities and therefore turns to theology and anthropology as a supplement to it. This approach builds on biblical depictions of God's covenantal relationship with human beings and emphasizes the freedom and autonomy of people to take responsibility for their lives, well-being, and environment in partnership with God. Like *"halakhic* formalism," the covenantal position also allows for a variety of substantive views within the system, and it too is transdenominational in its appeal.

Richard McCormick observes that the Catholic tradition can certainly provide guidance in dealing with mortal choices, but that guidance does not come in the form of ready-made solutions, answers, and conclusions. It comes rather as a theological framework that tells the redeeming story of Jesus Christ's life and example. It is that narrative which provides the insights, perspectives, and themes necessary for telling us who we are, where we are going, and what kind of people we ought to become. So, for example, for those who construe earthly life as a pilgrimage and not by itself our lasting home, claims by the State to have an unqualified interest or obligation in maintaining life-support for patients in a persistent vegetative state will not be supportable. Acknowledging that the Christian story is no longer widely functional in secular and pluralistic Western societies, he identifies a variety of moral problems that have followed from this fact. As alternatives to "reason without faith" and "reason replaced by faith," he closes by outlining the practical consequences of Catholicism's commitment to "reason informed by faith." These consequences include an appraisal of the relative status of life and death on the hierarchy of human goods and a policy that not all means should be used to preserve life. From this point the Catholic heritage leaves deliberations and decisions to those who must make them, but takes as its main task the nourishing of the decision-maker.

Concluding both this section and the volume itself, Martin Marty surveys a variety of problems that have made it difficult for religious heritages to establish clear links with ethics and medicine in a secular, democratic, and pluralistic age. Part of what it is to be modern, he contends, is to be jolted from living within a single tradition to at least an awareness of and perhaps an openness to a great variety of traditions and insights among which individuals can and often do feel an urgent need to choose. To draw guidance from a heritage, Marty argues that it is necessary first to recognize that we are in a tradition which conditions us, so that none of us really has access to the truth itself unconditioned by history. It is necessary further to take some possession of one's heritage by coming to know it well, lest by failing to do so, the heritage simply take possession of us. Using numerous examples drawn from the world's religions, he maintains that it is both easier and better to draw guidance from a heritage if there is a variety of competing views and interpretations of it than if there were only one system per culture, heteronomously imposed on its members. The reason is that the presence of many competing voices speaking about mortal choices necessitates that we cultivate habits of patient listening, broadened reflection, and critical appropriation of whatever clues our traditions offer about life and death. To the question of why we should even pay attention to what ancient religious heritages have to say, he answers that "they knew back there already what we do not know as yet." Thus, he concludes, by living in and observing communities that nourish and are nourished by a complex tradition, we may yet find options and possibilities that have long been overlooked.

Running through many of these discussions are a number of problematic issues that will call for much additional reflection by professionals and lay people concerned with bioethics. They include at least four main topics.

1. *The Challenge of Pluralism.* The great diversity of moral perspectives that characterizes modern liberal democracies provides an important impetus to moral reflection. At the same time, however, such diversity poses serious difficulties to reaching a moral consensus on issues that may genuinely require it. For example, is it possible to identify objective medical benefits when people living in a pluralistic society inevitably attach different meanings and evaluations to these same benefits? Can a strong commitment to pluralism and tolerance for differences accommodate an equally strong commitment to personal morality based on choice? Are moral disagreements within such a society necessarily irresolvable? Or are they only resolvable by political means that ultimately ignore the moral nature of the disagreements? Must the publicly accessible domain of moral consensus within such societies necessarily be a secular domain?

2. *Social Policy Decisions.* The costs and resources necessary for providing health care consistent with our values and moral traditions increasingly call for large-scale social policy decisions. Can bioethics illuminate the complex network of levels and relationships in health care delivery that will pose meaningful alternatives for making those decisions? Is it possible to decide what constitutes a decent or adequate level of health care? What special factors govern the allotment of health care resources as against other kinds of benefits in a modern democratic society? What, ultimately, should the aims of medicine be as a social enterprise?

3. *The Problem of Autonomy and the Common Good.* Personal autonomy is repeatedly depicted as being in tension, if not in conflict, with concern for the common good. What conceptions of autonomy contribute to conflict as opposed to only tension? What other principles are necessary to supplement the exercise of autonomy so that it does not become merely an egoistic expression of individual willfulness? Conversely, what other values and principles should supplement a concern for the common good so that it does not become a means for suppressing respect for persons and the value of individual choice?[6]

4. *The Relation of Thought and Practice.* The copious literature of contemporary bioethics has provided a remarkable range of insights into the

dilemmas that surround the development of modern medical practice and its reliance on new technologies. It has also offered a wide range of analyses and alternatives for resolving, or at least coping with, these dilemmas. How are these theoretical insights to be translated into the actual care of individuals? Can health care delivery be the same thing as treating patients? Is the subject matter of bioethical discussion a body of theory that can be "applied" to practice, or is it supposed to inform practice in a different way, through the reflectiveness of the practitioner? What models for integrating thought and practice exist now or could be developed to train increasingly specialized professionals to care for those who enter "the system"?[7]

The answers to these questions are by no means obvious. But their importance is generally recognized, and they surely call for both individual consideration and public discussion in our pursuit of better health. One thing, however, is certain. The way we choose to answer these questions and to live out the answers will decisively affect the character and quality of that precious time allotted to us all between our time to be born and our time to die.

Cincinnati, Ohio

NOTES AND REFERENCES

1.   R. B. Y. Scott, ed. and trans., *The Anchor Bible: Proverbs and Ecclesiastes* (Garden City, NY: Doubleday, 1965), 206.

2.   Francis Bacon, *The Advancement of Learning*, Book I, William A. Armstrong, ed., (London: The Athlone Press, 1975), 81. For more extended recent discussions of Bacon's project, see Jerry Weinberger, *Science, Faith, and Politics: Francis Bacon and the Utopian Roots of the Modern Age* (A Commentary on Bacon's *Advancement of Learning*) (Ithaca, NY: Cornell University Press, 1985), and Charles Whitney, *Francis Bacon and Modernity* (New Haven, CT: Yale University Press, 1986).

3.   Robert Hooke, *Micrographia* (London: The Royal Society, 1664), 7–8 (Preface). Reprinted with a Preface by R. T. Gunther (New York: Dover, 1961). Cf. Bacon, op. cit., 4–10, 26–27, 52–55.

4.   Recent statistics on changes in life expectancy in the United States provide a useful illustration of the problem of gain vs. loss in technological advances. Jacob A. Brody points out that "in 1900 only 25% of persons in the United States lived beyond age 65, while by 1985 approximately 70% survived age 65, and 30% lived to be 80 or more . . . . The central issue raised by increasing longevity is that of net gain in active functional years versus total years of disability and

dysfunction. Present data are weak but suggest that for each good, active functional year gained, we add about 3.5 compromised years." See Jacob A. Brody, *Annual Review of Public Health* 8 (1987): 211–212. I would like to thank Dr. Lynn Sommers of the University of Cincinnati School of Nursing for bringing this statistic to my attention.

5.   Daniel Callahan, "Shattuck Lecture-Contemporary Biomedical Ethics," *New England Journal of Medicine* 302 (May 29, 1980): 1228–1229.

6.   Current discussions of these and related questions may be found in Gerald Dworkin, *The Theory and Practice of Autonomy* (Cambridge: Cambridge University Press, 1988); John Christman, ed., *The Inner Citadel: Essays on Individual Autonomy* (Oxford: Oxford University Press, 1989); James F. Childress, "The Place of Autonomy in Bioethics," *Hastings Center Report* vol. 20, no. 1 (January/February 1990): 12–17, and George J. Agich, "Reassessing Autonomy in Long-Term Care," *Hastings Center Report* vol. 20, no. 6 (November/December 1990): 12–17.

7.   See Donald Schoen, *The Reflective Practitioner* (New York: Basic Books, 1983) and Leon R. Kass, "Practicing Ethics: Where's the Action?" *Hastings Center Report* vol. 20, no. 1 (January/February 1990): 5–12 for perceptive discussions of this issue.

I
SURVEYING CURRENT ISSUES

1

Mortal Choices Today: A Survey of the Moral Issues

Ruth Macklin

INTRODUCTION

Long before the advent of modern medical technology, moral issues involving birth and death were a major focus of philosophical and religious thought. Among the ancients, Hippocrates enjoined physicians not to assist patients in attempts at suicide or abortion,[1] while in the first century A.D. the Roman philosopher Seneca wrote: "the wise man will live as long as he ought, not as long as he can. . . . He always reflects concerning the quality, and not the quantity, of his life. . . . He holds that it makes no difference to him whether his taking-off be natural or self-inflicted, whether it comes later or earlier. . . . It is not a question of dying earlier or later, but of dying well or ill."[2]

In the eighteenth century, David Hume observed that "age, sickness, or misfortune may render life a burthen, and make it worse even than annihilation," thus condoning suicide.[3] In contrast, Immanuel Kant asserted that suicide is "abominable because God has forbidden it; . . . it is abominable in that it degrades man's inner worth below that of the animal creation."[4] Yet despite the fact that these ethical concerns have always been with us, recent scientific and technological advances have multiplied the moral issues.

As one example, we have new reproductive technologies, such as *in vitro* fertilization and cryopreservation, which give rise to questions about the ownership and disposition of frozen embryos. To take another example, soon after the arrival of AIDS, a deadly new infectious disease, the scientific capability of testing blood for evidence of HIV infection in people who had no clinical symptoms of AIDS produced myriad ethical problems. To mention only a few: the acceptability of routine screening of selected groups for HIV infection, dilemmas of confidentiality regarding those who test positive, and controversial public health measures, such as distributing clean needles to intravenous drug users, and isolating individuals, such as infected prostitutes, who pose a risk of harm to others.

A large variety of more mundane yet ominous developments are also worthy of attention, and with these I shall begin. The following three episodes occurred recently in the hospitals where I work.

In the first episode, a patient with amyotrophic lateral sclerosis (ALS, Lou Gehrig's disease) who was *not* terminally ill requested that she be removed from the ventilator to which she had been attached for 4 years. Marjorie Brown was alert and had been repeatedly evaluated by psychiatrists as having full decisional capacity and not suffering from clinical depression. She was completely paralyzed except for the ability to blink her eyes. After Ms. Brown requested removal of the ventilator, the physicians and nurses caring for her held a conference and concurred that her wish should be granted. They then sought advice and assistance from the hospital's ethics committee. A consulting team from the ethics committee met with the team caring for Ms. Brown, and then went to the bedside. The team reported back to the ethics committee, recounting their conversation with the patient, a conversation made excruciatingly difficult by the fact that she had to spell out each word in answer to questions by blinking her eyes once for "yes" and twice for "no" as her nurse pointed to letters of the alphabet on a piece of cardboard.

After a lengthy ethics committee meeting and proper documentation in the patient's chart, the request was made to hospital administration to remove the respirator. Perhaps it was a mistake to have the administration involved in the case, but by now it was too late. The administrator consulted hospital counsel, who reviewed the case and the steps taken so far. Eventually—after too long a wait, from the patient's point of view—hospital counsel granted permission to remove the life supports. Despite the permission and legal assurance of hospital counsel, usually a very conservative force in protecting a hospital from liability, the hospital administrator still resisted. Months had passed since Marjorie Brown had initiated her request, and at this point the ethics committee argued strongly that the patient's rights were being violated. Eventually the patient's wish was granted, but not without an unconscionable delay that caused great distress to the patient and her caregivers. It is important to note that the patient's family, her physicians and nurses, the ethics committee and even the hospital counsel were prepared to honor her request. It was a hospital administrator whose resistance prevented the exercise of the patient's right to refuse continued medical treatment.

There are still people who have ethical qualms, usually stemming from their religious convictions, about removing life supports from patients, even patients who are alert, have decisional capacity, and have experienced the burdens of the medical treatment they seek to have withdrawn. But the case of Marjorie Brown did not involve any such opposition on ethical or religious grounds. A hospital administrator, acting on reasons that were never made clear, succeeded in thwarting the patient's moral and legal right to refuse continued medical treatment.

The second case, which occurred in a different hospital, involved a patient with AIDS who was terminally ill, in extreme suffering as he deteriorated, and like the patient with ALS, requested removal of his ventilator. His physicians, members of the ethics consultation team, and other caregivers concurred. The patient requested that he be sedated with morphine so he would not be awake and alert when the artificial respiration was withdrawn. His physician was prepared to administer morphine to the patient and to remain at the bedside throughout the process, to assure the patient's peaceful passage from life to death. The doctor perceived his dual obligation to respect his patient's right to have medical treatment withdrawn, and at the same time to relieve the patient's suffering.

The hospital administrator, however, feared that the cause of death might then be the morphine—which suppresses respiration—instead of removal of the life supports. The administrator insisted that a court order be sought. The medical staff and the ethics consultation team were worried that despite the clear legal right of competent patients to refuse medical treatment, a trial court judge in the hospital's jurisdiction might refuse to honor the patient's request. The jurisdiction in which the hospital is located is known to have judges whose personal convictions about preserving life supersede their willingness to recognize legal precedents. The case was eventually resolved by an alliance between physician and patient, who together agreed that the patient would not be given the morphine in advance, but the physician would wait until manifest suffering was evident. This succeeded in convincing the administrator that the doctor would then be acting in his medical role of relieving the patient's suffering rather than as a "euthanizer" administering a lethal dose of morphine.

The third case differed in several respects. The patient was in a coma following an automobile accident, and was 3 months' pregnant. She was judged to have no reasonable likelihood of recovering her mental function, although she might live for years in the coma. The patient's mother, who had already granted informed consent for surgery on her incapacitated daughter, now requested an abortion. The hospital administration refused to allow the abortion to take place, although it was well within the legally permissible time limit and there was a physician ready and willing to do the abortion. These administrators had seen no problem in allowing the comatose patient's mother to grant consent for risky neurosurgery, yet they were unwilling to honor her request to abort a previable fetus in her daughter, who would never regain consciousness.

The hospital attorney refused to seek a court order on behalf of the hospital and insisted that the patient's mother be the one to initiate a court proceeding, if that was what she wished. As these deliberations and delays were occurring, the comatose patient was getting dangerously close to the point of fetal viability, a point at which the legal and possibly ethical concerns would loom as real barriers to procuring an abortion.

In whose interest was that action being thwarted? Although there are individuals in our society who proclaim that the fetus has a right to life, there was no one connected with this case making that moral claim on behalf of the fetus. A hospital administrator had assumed decision-making authority that overrode both an incapacitated patient's family and hospital physicians willing to comply with the family's request.

These three cases illustrate ways in which hospital "risk managers" and administrators regularly insert themselves between patients and their physicians, or thwart family members as surrogate decision-makers. Hospital administrators sometimes seek to prevent competent, adult patients from refusing burdensome treatment even when physicians concur with the patient's wish. They often insist that a court order be obtained whenever there is a shred of doubt (which almost always exists) about what the law says.

Do patients and their families have any recourse in situations such as these? In all three cases, hospital ethics committees were involved, but with no ultimate authority to act. Individuals who seek to exercise their rights as patients are rendered powerless when they confront stubborn or ignorant risk managers or hospital attorneys whose mission is often at odds with what is in the patient's best interest. Where it was once physicians who overtreated patients because they believed it was their moral obligation to continue therapy, it is now hospital administrators and risk managers who insist on overtreatment out of fear of liability.

EMPOWERING PATIENTS: TWO DECADES OF PROGRESS

In the past 20 years there have been some striking changes in the way medicine was practiced for centuries. No longer is the physician a "father figure" making decisions for patients without their knowledge and permission. No longer may a physician withhold a diagnosis of cancer from a patient without being criticized as "paternalistic"—presuming to know what is "best" for the patient. It is now illegal, as well as un-ethical, to conduct medical research without the informed consent of human subjects. Today, patients have *rights*.

Hippocrates, the Greek physician called the "Father of Medicine," admonished physicians to conceal most things from patients, turning their attention away from what is being done to them and revealing nothing of their future or present condition. This Hippocratic tradition reigned for over two thousand years. A study published in 1961 reported that almost 90% of physicians at that time withheld from their patients the fact that they had cancer. And as recently as 1971, an editorial in the *Journal of the American Medical Association* questioned the obligation of doctors to tell a patient with a fatal disease the truth. The editorial was entitled "Must the Physician Set Himself above Nature and Play Supergod?"

By now, however, much has changed. Patients' "right to know" their diagnosis and prognosis is widely recognized. When the 1961 study of what physicians tell cancer patients was redone in 1977, 98% reported that their general policy is to tell the patient. This does not mean that physicians have an obligation to inflict unwanted information on their patients. But it does mean that the patient—not the doctor—should be the one to judge when and how much information should be disclosed.

Even when it comes to life-sustaining treatments, most doctors have ceased to believe that they have an obligation to prolong a patient's life despite the patient's wishes. Both experienced physicians and recent graduates of medical school have, for the most part, come to respect their patients' right to participate in decisions surrounding their care, including the right to refuse life-prolonging treatment. Although many physicians still struggle with the proper balance between their obligation to do what they believe to be medically best for patients and their obligation to respect the patient's wishes, there are few doctors today who do not recognize their patients' right to participate in medical decision making.

Although this trend toward greater acceptance by doctors of their patients' role in decision making is not universal, it is notable. Moral progress cannot occur without a conception of an ideal for which to strive. That ideal is far from being fully attained in today's health care system, yet a greater recognition of patients' rights is a measure of progress toward that goal.

RATIONING MEDICAL CARE

The three cases described earlier illustrate one motive for hospital administrators, risk managers, or attorneys standing in the way of patients' or families' reasonable requests regarding treatment. The result in such cases is disenfranchisement of the legitimate and proper decision-makers, resulting in overtreatment of the patient.

Curiously, however, at the same time a different set of forces is at work that also removes patients from decision making. But it has the opposite effect on continuation of treatment. Attempts to implement "cost-containment" at the bedside, schemes to ration hospital care or medical treatment, limit the availability of therapy. When the items rationed are life-prolonging treatments or beds in an acute care hospital, neither patients nor their families have a say in whether life is to be prolonged.

A physician brought the following case to the hospital's ethics committee. The patient, about 70 years old, had been brought to the emergency room with a fever of 107° F. Following her admission to the hospital 7 months earlier, she was given a diagnosis of "status epilepticus." Now she is in the Intensive Care Unit, on a respirator from which she cannot be weaned. Brain damage is far-reaching. The doctors are having difficulty gaining access for the insertion of intravenous lines. The patient does not respond to stimuli, has already developed large decubitus ulcers (bedsores), and requires regular suctioning and turning. A private-duty nurse carries out these tasks of daily maintenance.

The patient's family—her husband and two daughters—were told of the bleak prognosis from the beginning. Yet they insist that this level of care be continued. The husband refuses to consider the physician's suggestion to write a "Do Not Resuscitate Order" for the patient. Contrary to expert medical evaluations, the family believes the patient is communicating with them. They refuse to believe the prognosis and hold out hope that the patient will recover.

In a number of ways, this case is not uncommon. Relatives of patients often demand treatment beyond the point where physicians are able to prevent death or restore functioning. Families sometimes maintain false hope—in their grief or denial—that a miracle will occur. Doctors are reluctant to ignore or override the wishes of a patient's family in such cases, not only out of fear of being sued but also out of respect for next of kin as surrogate decision-makers for patients who lack decisional capacity.

Yet there was a troubling aspect to this case, which was the reason the physician sought the help of the ethics committee. The doctor has been pressured by the hospital administration to discontinue this level of therapy because of financial costs. The hospital is paying for the private-duty nurse, and a bed in the ICU costs considerably more than one on a regular hospital floor. The patient is being given antibiotics, as well as artificial food and fluids, to maintain her life. The physician believes he should be an advocate for the family of his patient, and that the right course of action is to honor their wishes about the level of care being provided. Yet he is being criticized, even threatened, by his superiors for refusing to make financial considerations the overriding factor. The message is clear that this patient is absorbing a disproportionate share of the hospital's resources.

The physician told the ethics committee that the patient and her husband are Holocaust survivors, having spent years in a concentration camp. The family's experience under the Nazis underscores their unwillingness to forgo life-prolonging treatments. Some members of the ethics committee wonder whether it is ethically relevant that these people are Holocaust survivors. Everyone agrees that continued biological life could not benefit the patient herself. Yet some committee members are deeply worried about the justification for withdrawing treatment: the patient is costing the hospital too much money.

Today's trend to ration medical care clashes with the ongoing efforts of people who wish to play a role in their own treatment decisions. Furthermore, it holds the dangerous portent of judging certain lives to be not worthy of the cost it takes to maintain them, especially if costs are borne by the taxpayers. This has implications for social justice as well as for individual patients. It is likely to be poorer classes of patients, those on Medicaid and Medicare, whose continued care will prompt the question whether they are a "drain" on society.

If doctors accept a financial imperative to deliver less care, they consider it their obligation to engage in rationing at the bedside. A medical student, referring to an elderly, demented patient, asks: "Hasn't this patient cost society enough money already?" When physicians are urged or required to become society's fiscal gatekeepers, that is when they will cease to be advocates for their patients and begin instead to be their patients' adversaries.

The patients' rights movement of the past two decades arose in response to *over*treatment of patients by physicians who obeyed the technological imperative: "If it can be done, it must be done." Now the opposite danger has begun to emerge: *under*treating patients because treatment costs too much money. It is often said that "we all trust our own doctors." But will we continue to be able to do so in a system that has rendered physicians the servants of hospital administrators and insurance regulations?

PATIENT AGAINST PATIENT: COMPETITION
FOR SCARCE RESOURCES

It is true, nevertheless, that factors other than financial costs dictate the need to limit care provided to some patients. It is becoming increasingly common for patients to become competing rivals for scarce resources. Examples of truly scarce (in contrast to costly) resources are organs for transplantation, beds in critical care units, such as cardiac care and neonatal intensive care units, and specialized equipment in hospitals. Critical care units are almost always filled in hospitals, necessitating an allocation scheme for selecting patients. From an ethical point of view, the allocation should be one that is just. Adult critical care units typically engage in the practice of moving some patients out of a unit to make room for others. Patients falling into one of two groups might be moved: those well on the way to recovery, who will survive even if given a lower level of care; and those who are truly hopeless, who will die anyway even if kept in the ICU. A deeply troubling ethical problem exists when all patients who fit those criteria have already been moved out, and there are critically ill or injured patients in the emergency room awaiting admission to the ICU.

A peculiar situation arises in adult critical care units when potential patients—ones who have not yet appeared in the emergency room— loom as rivals for limited resources. A 77-year-old man was admitted to the emergency room of the hospital with acute chest pains. He came from a nursing home, was only slightly demented, and was a double amputee. Although information from the nursing home revealed that he had a son and a daughter, they did not accompany him nor did they visit at any time during his hospital stay. Repeated efforts were made to admit this patient to the Cardiac Care Unit, and the request was turned down each time. This was done in spite of the fact that there was an empty bed in the CCU. The director of the CCU gave these reasons for not admitting this patient: "Because of his age, dementia, and medical history, he's not a good candidate for the CCU." When asked about the empty bed, the director stated that it was standard practice to keep a bed in the unit open. "You never know who's going to show up later tonight."

Is it ethically justified to keep a bed open for this reason? The case would be clearer—at least to some observers—if there were another identified patient in competition with this patient for the last bed in the CCU. On whatever grounds a choice might be made between two actual patients in competition for a scarce resource, is there any basis for denying a bed to a patient already there when the competition is an unknown patient who has not yet arrived? When this case was presented, everyone suspected that the decision not to admit the elderly man was based more on a judgment of his quality of life and his social worth than on his medical prognosis. One participant commented: "If he had two legs instead of stumps, he would have been treated differently." Another person observed that if his son and daughter were present, demanding that "everything be done" for their father, the doctors would have reacted differently.

Questions of just allocation of resources occur prominently in the use of another life-saving technology—organ transplantation. Which principle of justice for distributing organs is most fair? The typical selection procedure is to move patients awaiting a heart transplant up the list when they become so sick they will die unless they are transplanted immediately. Yet one transplant surgeon has suggested that this procedure is unfair, as it fails to maximize the value of the donor heart.[5] A patient in less critical condition would come out of the operation healthier, and have a longer survival, thus making better use of the heart. In reply, opponents argue that it is unfair to those who have been on the list longer not to receive a transplant even if their prospects for survival are lower than the patient in competition for the organ.

Other hotly debated issues surrounding scarce organs for transplantation arise out of recent successes in liver transplants: How many livers is any one patient entitled to? Is it fair to patients on a list who have not received one attempted transplant to continue to wait while a patient who has had a failed transplant is given a second, third, or fourth chance? And what about alcoholics who have destroyed their liver by excessive drinking? Are they ethically entitled to have a transplant at all, while other patients with inherited liver disease remain on the list awaiting their turn?

There is probably no way to avoid situations in which life-saving resources that are truly limited, such as transplantable organs, pit one patient against another. The need exists to develop ethically sound criteria for allocating scarce medical resources. Beyond that, actual and proposed criteria should be made known to the public, instead of being used in secret by doctors and others responsible for distribution. Present and future patients have a right to know what criteria are employed and whether making exceptions is a common practice.

OTHER LIFE-THREATENING SITUATIONS

I contend that cost considerations should not be used at the bedside to limit the use of life-preserving treatment to patients. At the same time, limitations imposed by nature or circumstance require hard choices in the allocation of truly scarce resources. Are there other situations in which life-sustaining treatments may ethically be withheld from patients? One area of current controversy surrounds surgical replacement of heart valves in drug addicts who have infected their valves by repeated injections of drugs into their veins. In this situation, the replacement valves themselves are not a scarce resource, but the time of busy surgeons and other skilled health care professionals is a valuable resource.

Intravenous Drug Users with Infected Heart Valves

A cardiothoracic surgeon presented the following case at a recent meeting of the hospital ethics committee.

The patient was Derek Williams, a 38-year-old Vietnam veteran. Mr. Williams held a job, and had a wife and one child. He had been an intravenous drug user (IVDU) for years, with heroin as his drug of choice. His diagnosis was an infected aortic valve in his heart.

Williams had been a regular patient at a VA hospital in another borough of the city, and had had one valve replaced in March 1988. Following the surgery, he shot up again, and his prosthetic valve became infected in August of last year. He went back to the hospital where he had been treated, and an abscess was found around the valve. The patient was given a 1-month course of antibiotics and was discharged. Again he shot up, went back to the hospital, and allegedly was told: "You had your chance." Williams claims he was told to try one or two (named) private hospitals. When later questioned, personnel at the VA hospital denied having made that suggestion.

The surgeon presenting the case acknowledged some medical uncertainty about whether this was a failed cure of the past infection or a reinfection from shooting up again. He also wondered whether that mattered, with respect to his obligation to treat the patient.

Derek Williams was not now in heart failure, nor had he thrown a clot. But clinical assessment indicated the high likelihood that surgery would be necessary in 6 weeks, both to replace the newly infected valve and to repair the cavity resulting from the abscess.

Surgeons at the previous VA hospital where Williams had been seen were reported to have said: "We only operate once. Patients like this are not given a second chance. Although it's not written down anywhere, this is the unofficial policy. Resources are scarce, and we don't do a second valve replacement when the patient has reinfected a valve by shooting up."

The surgeon presenting the case noted three factors that make cure of the patient's immediate condition unlikely: the infection, the prosthesis, and the abscess. Does the likelihood of a negative outcome even if treatment is administered provide a good reason for denying the patient surgery? The surgeon reported that in a small series of patients having these characteristics, most came through the surgery reasonably well. So surgery could not reasonably be denied on medical grounds, in accordance with usual prognostic indications.

Now, however, the surgeon mentioned an additional complicating factor: Mr. Williams is HIV positive. He has no clinical signs of AIDS or AIDS Related Complex. Yet according to one medical view, repeated infections may be a beginning sign of immunodeficiency. Based on the experience of a San Francisco group, 30% of patients had developed full-blown AIDS in 5 years, and 50% in 10 years. Are these prognostic implications of HIV disease reasons for denying the patient surgery? Unless a patient is septic, with systemic disease caused by the presence of microorganisms or their toxins in the blood or tissues, the prognosis from HIV disease is not a contraindication for surgery.

So, the surgeon concluded, the real question is not Derek William's HIV infection, but rather his heroin addiction. The surgeon asked: "Can permanent addiction be considered a 'fatal condition'? Does a person who has had endocarditis have a 'fatal condition'?" This surgeon's experience, going back to 1978, has shown that all patients who were addicted and had endocarditis—with one exception—had died. Clinical experience demonstrates that the recalcitrant addict who has been operated on once ends up dying of his disease, *whether or not* another valve replacement is needed. So the prognostic indications for surgery based on Derek William's "disease" of intravenous drug addiction differ considerably from the prognostic indications stemming from his HIV infection.

To sort out the obligation of doctors toward intravenous drug users whose behavior has caused their heart valves to become infected requires some comparisons with other cases. Consider the case of a patient who is not a drug addict in need of surgery. Suppose the patient has incurable cancer that will cause her death in the same period of time that the drug addict's addiction will cause his death. The prognosis in terms of survival years would be the same. One difference is the patient's so-called "voluntary contribution" to his own disease. Is that consideration ethically relevant, from the standpoint of whether an obligation exists to perform surgery? A second potential difference is the possibility that the intravenous drug user might change his behavior, thus leading to a quite different prognosis.

Some argue that patients who have caused their own disease are not entitled to a share of scarce or expensive resources, including the time required for highly skilled surgeons to perform the operation, the care delivered by nursing staff, and a bed in the intensive care unit. Others claim that a patient's past health-risking behavior should not be taken into account in considering whether to treat them, but the likelihood of their continuing that pattern of behavior in the future should be a factor. Still others in this debate claim that patients' contribution to their own disease is not a morally relevant factor, and should never be used in determining whether treatment should be administered.

An analogous context in which a similar debate has raged was mentioned earlier: liver transplantation for alcoholics who have destroyed their livers by excessive alcohol consumption. Criteria used by leading transplant surgeons to select patients for a liver transplant do *not* automatically rule out as candidates alcoholics who have destroyed their livers by drinking. According to one transplant surgeon, the focus should lie in "medical appropriateness": "if one could transplant livers in alcoholics with a reasonable minimal success rate, it is appropriate."[6] Instead of adopting a "backward-looking" criterion for exclusion—the past health-risking behavior of the patient—transplant surgeons say they employ a "forward-looking" criterion. A patient in need of a liver transplant who has remained abstinent from alcohol for a requisite period of time, and has undergone psychological assessment, could be on a list to receive a liver transplant.[7]

Using this approach to drug addicts, abstention from intravenous drugs would qualify past drug users with infected valves to receive surgery. Skeptics will no doubt argue that addicts might be able to remain drug-free during that waiting period, but as soon as the surgery is performed, they will return to their old habits. That is an empirical question, one that can be answered only by gathering relevant data.

There appears to be a nationwide trend in which cardiac surgeons are not doing repeat valve operations. Many avoid trying to do the surgery on such patients following the first infection. According to the surgeon who presented the case of Derek Williams, some hospitals in Miami have agreed to share the addicts: each will do one valve replacement, and no hospital will do a second operation.

The surgeon concluded by asking: "What about the patient who is found taking drugs while still in the hospital, through an intravenous line? Should that patient be given a repeat operation if his valve becomes reinfected?" Most ethics committee members agreed that this would be the limiting case, but their conclusion seemed to be based on their feelings about drug addicts and their antisocial behavior rather than on a principled moral argument.

This was not the first instance of such cases being brought to our hospital ethics committee. In fact, this same surgeon had brought a similar case to the meeting of a committee at another affiliated hospital. His position had once been that performing these operations was not medically contraindicated. Furthermore, he had refused to view drug addicted patients as "guilty" of causing their own disease and, therefore, not deserving of treatment. But he was being worn down by his surgical colleagues. Increasingly, he stood alone as one who believed there was an obligation to treat. He now brings these cases to the ethics committee for additional guidance, to see whether the committee shares the position held by an apparent majority of surgeons. Committee members were divided on the issue.

Maternal–Fetal Conflict

This brief survey of mortal choices in today's medical world has focused so far on the end of life, revealing different sources of moral problems. Technological advances, such as the ability to transplant organs, replace infected heart valves, and provide life-prolonging intensive care create dilemmas of justice in allocating resources. Managerial concerns about the cost of medical treatment and the prospect of legal liability diminish the authority of physicians and intrude into the doctor-patient relationship. Before concluding, let me turn to the beginning of life and address a recent issue that has come to be known as "maternal–fetal conflict."

Medicine's enhanced diagnostic capabilities, including the use of fetal assessment tools, is one factor that has contributed to a situation in which a pregnant woman and her fetus can become adversaries, with rights and interests in conflict. In addition, the deep societal problem of drug and alcohol abuse includes pregnant women whose behavior risks the health of their future children. The result has been a growing tendency to control pregnant women for the sake of the fetus or for the child that fetus will become.

Physicians have recommended and sought to impose a number of different medical or surgical interventions on pregnant women, sometimes for their own benefit but usually for the sake of the fetus. Perhaps the most common of these is cesarean section, which women have refused on religious grounds, because of fear of cutting, or for other reasons—some rational, others irrational. It should be recalled, however, that adult, competent patients with decisional capacity have a legal and moral right to refuse medical treatment, even if their reason for refusing is thought to be irrational. A pregnant woman may be forced to take medication, such as penicillin, for the sake of fetal health. In a case that occurred in 1982, a court ordered a pregnant, diabetic woman to receive insulin treatment despite her refusal on religious grounds.[8] Going back many years, Jehovah's Witnesses have been compelled to receive unwanted blood transfusions, including transfusions performed well before the onset of fetal viability. In a case that occurred in Jamaica Hospital in New York in 1985, a court ordered a Jehovah's Witness to be transfused when the fetus was only 18 weeks in gestation.[9]

In addition to recommending and obtaining legal coercion for specific medical interventions, physicians have recently sought more generally to compel a woman's compliance during pregnancy. "Doctor's orders" have included putting on weight or limiting weight gain, eating particular foods, taking vitamins and other medications, not carrying heavy groceries, making and keeping doctor's appointments,[10] and refraining from having sexual relations.

Most recently, there has been a strong movement joined by physicians, prosecutors, legislators and others to coerce, incarcerate, or indict as criminals women who use drugs or abuse alcohol during pregnancy. This movement is not confined to the use of illegal substances, since alcohol is perfectly legal but, as is well known, can cause problems for an infant as bad as or even worse than various illegal substances.

Universal agreement can be attained on the proposition that pregnant women have a *moral* obligation to act in ways likely to result in the birth of a sound, healthy infant. Yet views about what follows from this proposition differ sharply. The list of points about which there is debate or disagreement includes at least the following:

1. The pregnant woman's moral obligation should (or should not) be construed as an obligation to the fetus *in utero*.
2. The pregnant woman's moral obligation should (or should not) be transformed into a legal obligation.
3. The pregnant woman's obligation gives rise (or fails to give rise) to a corresponding right, either of the fetus *in utero* or the future child the fetus is likely to become.
4. The pregnant woman has (or does not have) an inviolable right to be free from coercive intrusions or invasions into her body, her liberty, or her privacy.
5. The fetus does (or does not have) moral standing.
6. There should (or should not be) an immoral act or a crime termed "fetal abuse."

None of these points follows directly from the claim that pregnant women have a moral obligation to act in ways likely to result in the birth of a sound, healthy infant. Additional premises are needed to yield any of these conclusions, as well as other controversial statements about the rights and interests of pregnant women, embryos, fetuses, and future children.

What follows from the view that pregnant women have an obligation toward their future children? Like other moral obligations, this one is contingent on a reasonable ability to comply. This stems from the philosophical precept "ought implies can"—before people can be assigned moral obligations to act or refrain from acting in certain ways, it must be physically and psychologically possible for them to act in those ways. What constitutes a "reasonable ability to comply" with a moral obligation is often uncertain and open to dispute. In the case of pregnant women, a number of different constraints might limit their ability to comply with the obligation to act in ways that promote the health of their future children.

If the woman is a heroin addict, she may not have access to a treatment program. If she is an alcoholic, she may have tried—and failed— to combat her alcoholism. If she is a crack addict, her addiction might overpower her wish to do what is best for her future infant, in light of the fact that there is no currently effective treatment for cocaine addiction. If she is a Jehovah's Witness, the strength of her religious belief may preclude her accepting a blood transfusion recommended for the well-being of the fetus. She might refuse surgical intervention out of religious convictions, an overwhelming fear of cutting, or having experienced a relative's death from an anesthesia accident. If she has been advised by her obstetrician late in pregnancy not to have sexual intercourse, she may be unable to resist her husband's insistence out of fear of violence on his part. These or other circumstances can lead to legitimate questions about a pregnant woman's reasonable ability to carry out her obligation to promote the health of her future child. The "ought implies can" maxim requires an assessment of each case or circumstance to determine whether the obligation is one that the woman is capable of fulfilling.

Nevertheless, the moral obligation is presumed to exist in the absence of evidence to the contrary. However, pregnant women's moral obligation to promote the health of their infants should *not* be transformed into a legal obligation. Not everything that is immoral should also be made illegal. Some actions are morally wrong, yet are not made subject to the force of law.

Furthermore, legal coercion of pregnant women is too strong a response to their behavior, given that (1) competent adults have a moral and legal right to refuse medical interventions that place them at risk; (2) standards for taking away people's liberty by incarcerating them should be based on actual, serious harms already committed or a high probability of serious future harm to another existing person; and (3) social injustice is highly likely because of the greater numbers of poor and minority women who will be suspected, reported, or indicted for the alleged "crime" of fetal abuse.

One price of upholding individual liberty in a free society is the occurrence of some tragic birth defects and impaired children. Although some tragedies are preventable, it is ethically unacceptable to seek to maximize prevention through legal coercion of the sort proposed and in some cases actually carried out with pregnant women. To seek to prevent some tragic illnesses and infant deaths by erecting a system that pits physician against patient makes criminals out of women who risk the health of their future children. It requires that women be sedated and strapped down to undergo cesarean sections or blood transfusions, which is both desperate and extreme. The conclusion appears inescapable: a balance of *bad* consequences over good, both for women and for society generally, is more likely to result if legal coercion of pregnant women is endorsed.

CONCLUSION

This survey of today's moral issues surrounding birth and death reveals that they remain controversial, provoking disagreements among reasonable people who embrace different religious or philosophical positions. Although we may never come to universal agreement or reach a consensus on many of these moral issues, we can all profit from a clear understanding of where and why we disagree. My aim in this survey has been to provide some clarity toward that end.

NOTES AND REFERENCES

1.   Oath of Hippocrates. See *Encyclopedia of Bioethics*, Vol. 4 (New York: The Free Press, 1978), 1731.

2.   Seneca, *Epistula Morales*, Vol. 2, reprinted in *Moral Problems in Medicine*, 2nd ed. Samuel Gorovitz and Ruth Macklin *et al.*, eds., (Englewood Cliffs, NJ: Prentice-Hall, 1983), 433.

3.   David Hume, "Essay on Suicide," reprinted in S. Gorovitz and R. Macklin, 437–442.

4.   Immanuel Kant, "Suicide," reprinted in S. Gorovitz and R. Macklin, 437.

5.   O. Jonasson, "Waiting in Line: Should Selected Patients Ever Be Moved Up?" *Transplantation Proceedings*, 21, 3 (June 1989): 3390–3394.

6.   A. P. Monaco, "Roundtable Discussion: Patient Selection Criteria in Organ Transplantation: The Critical Questions," *Transplantation Proceedings*, 21, 3 (June 1989): 3416.

7.   This point was made at a Conference on Patient Selection Criteria in Transplantation: The Critical Questions, March 14–15, 1989, Ann Arbor, Michigan.

8.   Nancy K. Rhoden, "Informed Consent in Obstetrics: Some Special Problems," *Western New England Law Review*, 9 (1987): 82.

9.   *Ibid.*

10.   Martha A. Field, "Controlling the Woman to Protect the Fetus," *Law, Medicine, & Health Care*, 17 (Summer 1989): 115.

2

Birth, Death, and the Criminal Law: The New Politics of Privacy

George J. Annas

For the past two decades Americans have been involved in a highly vocal, and sometimes violent, debate about the role of the criminal law in regulating decisions made at the beginning and end of life. With notable exceptions such as Vonnegut's "Welcome to the Monkey House," and Hitler's Germany, issues regarding pregnancy and birth have seemed irrelevant to issues involving death. For example, the struggle over abortion rights has seldom been directly linked to the dying patient, and the term "euthanasia" has seldom been seen as relevant to abortion. Nonetheless, issues concerning birth and death are intimately linked because both involve decisions that powerfully impact on one's view of self, and are inseparable from any coherent view of human dignity. In the United States, the code word we have used to describe personal decisions that the government should generally not interfere with is "privacy."

Two examples illustrate the new politics of privacy. On July 3, 1989, the day the United States Supreme Court decided the controversial abortion case in *Webster*,[1] the Court agreed to hear the appeal of Nancy Cruzan, a woman in a persistent vegetative state whose parents wanted tube feeding discontinued. A later front page headline in the *New York Times* properly tied the issues in both cases together: "High Court Facing Fight on Abortion, Privacy and Death."[2]

The second item was much less publicized, but dramatically portrays the political potential of linking issues of birth and death together. In early November 1989, John Cardinal O'Connor of New York proposed establishing a new order of nuns, called the "Sisters of Life," who would be specifically dedicated to ending abortion and mercy killing. These

35

nuns, whose members would include lawyers and physicians, would not only pray and work directly with the elderly, poor, and sick, but would also be heavily involved in legislative lobbying. In Cardinal O'Connor's words: "Because we are such a litigious society and there are so many new laws being proposed in Congress and the state legislatures, we need people who will devote full-time to keeping up with the law and who will say, 'This is what we believe.'"[3]

What is the role of the criminal law at the beginning and end of life? Surely it has a proper role in protecting the sanctity of life and in protecting the weak from the strong. But the limits of the criminal law in this context have always been problematic. As Glanville Williams, the noted British medicolegal scholar, wrote more than three decades ago in introducing his classic study of the subject:

> Law has been called the cement of society, and certainly society would fall to pieces if men could murder with impunity. Yet there are forms of murder, or near-murder, the prohibition of which is rather the expression of a philosophical attitude than the outcome of social necessity. These are infanticide, abortion, and suicide. Each extends the disapprobation of murder to particular situations which raise special legal, moral, religious, and social problems.[4]

Legal jurisprudential expert, Lon Fuller has suggested that we can gain useful insights into the areas in which criminal law can play a constructive role in society by distinguishing between "the morality of aspiration and the morality of duty."[5] The morality of aspiration, he says, is exemplified in Greek philosophy, "the morality of the Good Life, of excellence, of the fullest realization of human powers." On the other hand, the morality of duty "starts at the bottom [and] . . . lays down the basic rules without which an ordered society is impossible . . . it condemns for failing to respect the basic requirements of social living." In the United States, the debate on where the criminal law line should be drawn between "aspiration" and "duty" has become embodied in the debate on the right of privacy, and it is on the contours of the constitutional right of privacy that this paper concentrates.

The United States government is based on the Constitution, and the Amendments to the Constitution restrict the power of both the federal and state governments to make laws dealing with certain areas of fundamental individual rights (or liberty), such as free speech, freedom of religion, and freedom of association. Therefore, the interpretation of the Constitution as it applies to individual liberty in the areas of birth and death will determine what areas, if any, are beyond majoritarian rule. Areas not so protected are fair game for the legislative process, and thus for the criminal law. Since many, if not most, birth and death decisions will be made in the context of a doctor-patient relationship, the ultimate contours of the right of privacy will also have profound implications for the practice of medicine in the United States.

CONSTITUTIONAL ISSUES IN MEDICINE

Neither the word "medicine" nor the word "health" appears in the Constitution, and the federal government itself has no direct authority in these areas. The state governments retained sovereignty, and with it the inherent "police powers" to legislate to protect the public's health, safety, and morals. The federal government gets authority in these areas only indirectly, primarily through its power to tax and spend, to regulate interstate commerce, and to provide for the national defense.

When either the state or federal government legislates in the area of medicine, it is bound by limitations set forth in the Bill of Rights and the other Amendments to the Constitution that restrict the actions the government can take by protecting certain individual rights of citizens. The most prominent of these rights has come to be designated the "right of privacy." Although this right does not explicitly appear in the text of the Constitution, the Court has found it implicit in the "concept of personal liberty" embodied in the Fourteenth Amendment. It can properly be described as a right to be "left alone" with at least three aspects: (1) *informational* (a right to have certain private information kept private); (2) *territorial* (a right to have certain private places, like one's bedroom, free from government intrusion); and (3) *personal* (a right to make certain private decisions free from government interference). The third is the one most directly involved in a growing notion of the right to control one's body. The question is how much control an individual should have when seemingly personal decisions affect the community. Stated in constitutional terms, assuming a personal decision is properly viewed as protected by the "right of privacy," when can the state nonetheless demonstrate a "compelling interest" in regulating or prohibiting it? Rephrased in broader terms the overarching question is: Which birth and death decisions should be left in the realm of morality, and which should be regulated by the criminal law?

DECISION MAKING AT THE BEGINNING OF LIFE

The most notorious case involving human reproduction was decided by the U.S. Supreme Court in 1927. In it the Court upheld the constitutionality of a Virginia statute that permitted, among other things, the involuntary sterilization of the "feeble-minded." Justice Oliver Wendell Holmes wrote for the Court:

> It is better for all the world, if instead of waiting to execute degenerate offspring for crime, or let them starve for their imbecility, society can prevent those who are manifestly unfit from continuing their kind. . . . Three generations of imbeciles are enough.[6]

This case capped three decades of the eugenics movement in the United States and was heavily influenced by it. It suggested constitutional support for a movement to limit the right to procreate to those with sufficiently high IQs. It was not until 15 years later that the Court again examined the issue. This time it struck down an Oklahoma statute that provided for the compulsory sterilization of "habitual criminals." It applied to larceny, but specifically exempted persons convicted of embezzlement. The eugenics movement had fallen into disfavor, and the Court was more willing to look at the rights of the individuals involved. Justice William Douglas, writing for the Court, ruled that the statute violated the equal protection clause of the Fourteenth Amendment, and along the way affirmed the fundamental "value of reproductive autonomy over a majoritarian decision in favor of sterilization." In the Court's words:

> We are dealing here with legislation which involves one of the basic civil rights of man. *Marriage and procreation are fundamental to the very existence and survival of the race.* The power to sterilize, if exercised, may have subtle, far-reaching and devastating effects. In evil or reckless hands, it can cause races or types which are inimical to the dominant group to wither and disappear.[7]

Even though *Buck v. Bell* has never been explicitly overturned, the vast majority of commentators believe it is no longer good law, and that at the very least the Court would require a high level of procedural protection before any involuntary sterilization would be permissible. One approach, approved by the New Jersey Supreme Court, is that involuntary sterilization is impermissible unless a court finds, by clear and convincing evidence, that it is in the person's best interests. Among the factors the court must consider in reaching this conclusion are the existence of technological alternatives such as contraception, and even if sterilization is approved, use of the least drastic means to accomplish it (e.g., tubal ligation instead of hysterectomy).[8]

Both contraception and abortion have been highly regulated and even outlawed when society viewed them as immoral. Both the changing mores of society and the development of effective oral contraceptives and a safe and effective means of first trimester abortion (suction aspiration) have strongly influenced the Court's views on the constitutional rights of individuals to use these technologies. The Supreme Court's premier decision on contraception, in which the Court enunciated the "right of privacy" for the first time in the reproduction context, was heard shortly after oral contraception became popular in the United States.

In that 1965 case, *Griswold* v. *Connecticut*,[9] the Court found a Connecticut statute that forbade the use of contraceptives unconstitutional as a violation of the "zones of privacy" that surround sexual relations in marriage. Seven years later, the Court determined that it was the sexual relationship and the potential to produce a child that was critical, not the marriage itself, so that a statute that only prohibited nonmarried individuals from using contraception was unconstitutional as well.[10] In the Court's words, "If the right to privacy means anything, it is the right of the individual, married or single, to be free from unwarranted governmental intrusions into matters so fundamentally affecting a person as the decision whether to bear or beget a child." The final, and most contentious, series of cases deal with abortion, a question on which Americans remain deeply ambivalent.[11]

Roe v. Wade

In the 1973 case of *Roe* v. *Wade*,[12] and all the abortion cases that have followed it (other than those about financing abortion), the Supreme Court has been faced with a criminal statute designed to limit access to abortion. In *Roe*, the Texas statute the Court was reviewing made it a crime to procure an abortion or to attempt one, except to save the life of the mother. Justice Harry Blackmun, former legal counsel to the Mayo Clinic, wrote the opinion of the Court. One of his major personal goals in writing the opinion was to prevent the government from interfering with the practice of medicine and the doctor-patient relationship.[13]

The decision was seven to two, with Justices William Rehnquist and Byron White dissenting. The Court determined that a fundamental right of privacy existed "in the Fourteenth Amendment's concept of personal liberty and restrictions upon state action." The Court went on to hold that this fundamental right "is broad enough to encompass a woman's decision whether or not to terminate her pregnancy":

> The detriment that the State would impose upon the pregnant woman by denying this choice altogether is apparent. Specific and direct harm medically diagnosable even in early pregnancy may be involved. Maternity, or additional offspring, may force upon a woman a distressful life and future. Psychological harm may be imminent. Mental and physical health may be

taxed by child care. . . . . All these are factors the woman and her responsible physician necessarily will consider in consultation.

Although granting decisions about abortion a very high degree of constitutional protection, the Court stopped short of declaring that a woman's right to an abortion was absolute or that she had a right to an abortion on demand. Instead the Court recognized that the state also had interests that might at times be compelling enough to limit abortion. The Court identified two such interests: the protection of maternal health and the protection of viable fetuses. The protection of maternal health has always been a legitimate interest of the state. The Court ruled, however, that this interest could never be compelling enough to prohibit abortion before the stage of pregnancy when it is less dangerous for the woman to carry the fetus to term than to have an abortion (which in 1973 was about the end of the first trimester). The Court decided that during the first trimester the state could regulate abortions to protect the woman's health only by requiring that they be performed by a physician. Thereafter it could regulate abortions to protect women only in ways reasonably calculated to enhance their personal health, rather than in ways designed to protect the fetus or simply to discourage abortions.

The second state interest the Court identified was that of "protecting the potentiality of human life." The Supreme Court did not decide that a fetus is not human, only that a fetus is not a "person" as that term is used in the Fourteenth Amendment. The Court also noted that "the pregnant woman cannot be isolated in her privacy"; her interests in privacy must be weighed against the state's interest in the life of the fetus. The question is: When does the state's interest become so compelling that the state can justifiably interfere with a woman's constitutional right to have an abortion? No satisfactory answer to this question can be garnered from science, and any demarcation during pregnancy is inherently arbitrary.[14] The Court decided to choose the point of fetal viability—the point at which the fetus "is potentially able to live outside the mother's womb, albeit with artificial aid"—as the demarcation, apparently because at this point the fetus is biologically identical to a premature infant.

After viability, which continues to occur near the end of the second trimester, varying somewhat with medical advances and skill, the state "may, if it chooses, regulate, and even proscribe, abortion except where it is necessary, in appropriate medical judgment, for the preservation of the life or health of the mother." Although states can regulate abortions after fetal viability (or, more accurately, can restrict the induction of premature birth), since *Roe* only 13 states have enacted laws to restrict such abortions.[15]

In more than a dozen major cases over the succeeding 15 years, the Supreme Court applied *Roe* to specific attempts by some states to limit abortion rights during the first and second trimesters. Until 1989, the Court consistently struck down almost all such limitations. The Court did find it constitutional, however, for the state and federal governments to refuse to fund abortions through the Medicaid program because, in the Court's view, the failure to finance abortions did not place a governmental obstacle in the path of a woman who wanted to terminate her pregnancy.[16] The Court also ruled that states could properly mandate general informed consent requirements, confidential recordkeeping and reporting related to maternal health, pathological examination of fetal tissue, and the presence of a second physician when a pregnancy was terminated after fetal viability.[17] In the Court's view, none of these requirements limits a woman's ability to choose an abortion or a physician's ability to perform one.

Regulations that the Court rejected as unconstitutional under *Roe* included those giving the husband or father veto power over the woman's decision, requiring that specific and detailed information concerning fetal development be given to the woman, and mandating hospitalization. By the mid-1980s the Court had made the precise boundaries of *Roe* very clear.[18]

Perhaps because the Supreme Court had been so consistent in upholding and expanding the rights recognized in *Roe*, opposition to the opinion continued. One's position on abortion rights became the litmus test in judicial appointments. Under President Ronald Reagan, who said he considered abortion "murder," judges were appointed to the U.S. Supreme Court who were openly opposed to the *Roe* v. *Wade* decision. By 1989, three Reagan appointees—Sandra Day O'Connor, Antonin Scalia, and Anthony Kennedy—had joined the two dissenters in *Roe*, who were still on the Court, and the possibility that a five-justice majority might retreat from *Roe* v. *Wade* or overrule it entirely first appeared. Both sides in the abortion rights debate were therefore hopeful or fearful of the Court's decision in *Webster*, and more friend-of-the-court briefs were filed in that case than in any other in the history of the United States.

The Webster Decision

In delivering its July 1989 opinion in *Webster*,[19] the Supreme Court reopened the national debate about the proper role of state governments in determining when abortions may take place within their borders, although technically the Court made no changes in *Roe* at all. At issue in *Webster* was a Missouri abortion statute that had 20 provisions. Because of the way the case was argued, the Court ruled on only three of them.

The Court ruled that Missouri could constitutionally prohibit state-employed physicians from performing an abortion that was not necessary to save the life of a woman, could prohibit such an abortion from being performed in state facilities, and could require physicians to attempt to determine fetal viability at or after 20 weeks' gestation.

None of these statutory restrictions is inconsistent with *Roe*, although the first two, like the earlier Medicaid funding decisions, will make it more difficult for poor women to obtain abortions. If this technical holding had been the only result of the case, it would have occasioned almost no comment. *Webster* is so important because five of the justices, writing three separate opinions, made it clear that they no longer believe the trimester scheme of *Roe* is tenable, and four of them are ready to permit states to regulate heavily, and perhaps even prohibit outright, most abortions at any point in pregnancy.

Roe v. *Wade* was based on two conceptual foundations: first, that there is a fundamental constitutional right of privacy broad enough to encompass a woman's decision to have an abortion; and second, that the state's interests in abridging the exercise of this right are related to the stage of pregnancy. The plurality opinion in *Webster* (on which only three justices agreed) ignored the right of privacy altogether. Although the scope of the constitutional right of privacy was the issue on which most friends of the court argued this abortion case, the Court did not seek to limit that right in areas other than abortion. As the American Medical Association properly noted in its own brief on *Webster*, the constitutional right of privacy (in the doctor-patient context) "simply reflects the historic tradition, embodied in our common law, of recognizing that all medical treatment decisions ordinarily should be made by the patient, after consultation with a physician concerning the risks and benefits of treatment."[20]

Instead the plurality concentrated exclusively on *Roe's* trimester scheme. The plurality said, for example, that "the key elements of the *Roe* framework—trimesters and viability—are not found in the text of the Constitution." The plurality concluded that rather than having to balance the rights of the individual and the interests of the state, states have a compelling interest "in protecting human life throughout pregnancy." If this is true, of course, then the fact that women have a fundamental constitutional right to decide to have an abortion does not help them in a state that outlaws abortion to protect fetal life, since compelling state interests trump individual rights.

Four justices indicated that they would uphold any restriction on abortion that "permissibly furthers the State's interest in protecting potential human life." Four others would continue to uphold the balance required by *Roe*. The ninth, Justice O'Connor, can create a five-to-four majority by joining either side of the debate. She had indicated her displeasure with the trimester scheme before *Webster* was decided, and she suggested that the Court determine the constitutionality of state abortion laws on the basis of whether they "unduly burden" a woman's right to an abortion.[21] But because she believed that the three provisions of the Missouri law were consistent with *Roe*, she refused to use *Webster* to reverse or restrict *Roe*.

Constitutional law regarding abortion thus remains the same after *Webster* as it was before. On the other hand, anyone who can count knows that one more change in the Supreme Court's membership, or a shift in Justice O'Connor's thinking, may result in the reversal of *Roe* and the granting of wide powers to state governments to restrict abortions.

The *Webster* decision has led to abortion becoming one of the most important issues in state-wide elections (and it played the key role in electing governors in New Jersey and Virginia in 1989). President George Bush has also made one's position on abortion a litmus test for high offices in the Department of Health and Human Services—a political loyalty test that has meant that as of the end of November 1989, almost a year into his presidency, President Bush has been unable to fill the positions of Director of the National Institutes of Health and Director of the Centers for Disease Control. The president has said, however, that he does favor the option of abortion following rape or incest, but has consistently vetoed congressionally approved legislation to fund abortions in cases of rape or incest for poor women under state, or the District of Columbia Medicaid programs. The abortion debate continues at all levels of government, and in the judiciary. The debate is newer, and less acrimonious, at the other end of life.

LEGAL LIMITS ON DECISION MAKING AT THE END OF LIFE

Unlike the abortion debate, which pits slogans like "the right to life" against slogans like "the right to choice," the debate on using medical technologies to delay death has focused mostly on individual stories, which can be seen as parables. The most famous such story is that of Karen Ann Quinlan.

The Case of Karen Ann Quinlan

Following an episode still incompletely understood, Ms. Quinlan was rushed to an emergency room and resuscitated (she had stopped breathing for at least 15 minutes). She never regained consciousness, but retained brain activity. Her breathing was done by a mechanical ventilator, and she was diagnosed as being in a persistent vegetative state—

essentially a permanent coma, in which one has sleep–wake cycles, but is totally unaware of one's environment or existence.

Convinced that their daughter's case was hopeless, her parents asked that the ventilator be removed so that she could die in peace. Her physicians were sympathetic, but fearing possible criminal prosecution for homicide, they insisted that her parents obtain a court order immunizing them from any legal liability should they discontinue the ventilator. The lower court refused, noting that the physicians who testified thought ventilator removal under the circumstances was unethical. The Supreme Court of New Jersey, in a landmark, unanimous decision, written by Chief Justice (and former Governor) Richard Hughes, reversed and authorized the removal on the basis of Ms. Quinlan's constitutional right of privacy, as the U.S. Supreme Court had articulated it in *Roe* v. *Wade*. In the court's words:

> It is the issue of the constitutional right of privacy that has given us most concern in the exceptional circumstances of this case. . . . Presumably this right is broad enough to encompass a patient's decision to decline medical treatment under certain circumstances, in much the same way as it is broad enough to encompass a woman's decision to terminate pregnancy under certain conditions.[22] (citing *Roe* v. *Wade*)

Having arrived at this sweeping conclusion with almost no analysis, and having distinguished a case only 5 years previously decided in which it had ruled that there is "no constitutional right to die" (on the basis that the young woman in that case was unable to express her wishes and was "apparently salvable to long life and vibrant health"[23]), the court went on to determine whether the state could demonstrate any "compelling interests" to prevent Karen Quinlan (or her guardian, acting on her behalf) from exercising her constitutional right to refuse medical treatment.

The court examined four possible interests: the preservation and sanctity of human life, prevention of suicide, protection of innocent third parties, and upholding the ethical integrity of the medical profession. The court found third parties irrelevant (since Ms. Quinlan had no dependents), and the ethics of the profession consistent with removal. The tougher issues were homicide and suicide. As to homicide, the court concluded that the ensuing death would be "from existing natural causes" and thus not homicide. And even if it was homicide, it would be justifiable homicide because it was "pursuant to the right of privacy." Suicide or "self-murder" is not a crime anywhere in the United States, but assisted suicide is. However, since there would be no homicide prosecution, there could also be no assisted suicide prosecution.

The *Quinlan* case has become the touchstone all other post-1976 courts have used in examining the reach of the constitutional "right of privacy" to refuse medical interventions. Some courts have based their decisions to permit treatment withdrawal on common law battery principles, but most have also followed *Quinlan* in enunciating a constitutional right to refuse treatment as well. Some have been more persuasive in arguing that the state really cannot show any compelling interest in forcing continued medical treatment on a competent individual. For example, the Massachusetts Supreme Judicial Court (SJC) has argued (in language that could equally be applied to abortion decisions) that honoring the right of privacy is itself honoring the sanctity of life:

> The constitutional right to privacy, as we conceive it, is an expression of the sanctity of individual free choice and self-determination as fundamental constituents of life. The value of life as so perceived is lessened not by a decision to refuse treatment, but by the failure to allow a competent human being the right to choice.[24]

As to suicide, the SJC noted that suicide required "irrational self-destruction," and could not exist unless the individual had *both* the intent to die and personally put the death-producing agent into motion with this intent. Death from natural causes would thus never qualify.

Since then, the supreme courts in both New Jersey and Massachusetts, and others, have determined that the constitutional right of privacy extends to refusing *any* medical intervention, including artificial feeding. The most notable exception to this line of cases is the case of Nancy Cruzan, currently before the U.S. Supreme Court. (See *addendum*.)

The Case of Nancy Cruzan

On a clear, cool January night in 1983, Nancy Cruzan, then 25 years old, was driving alone on a Missouri country road when, for reasons unknown, she drove off the road and was hurled from her car. She was found lying face down in a ditch, not breathing and apparently dead. Paramedics arrived, commenced CPR, and spontaneous respiration was restored after about 10 minutes. Nancy has never regained consciousness, and is currently maintained by a gastrostomy tube in a permanently unconscious condition at the Mt. Vernon State Hospital.

Nancy Cruzan's parents were appointed her guardians in January 1984. There is no material dispute about her medical condition. She is in a persistent vegetative state; she is oblivious to her environment except for reflexive responses to sound and "perhaps" painful stimuli; her cerebral cortical atrophy is irreversible, permanent, progressive, and ongoing. She cannot move her body, and will never recover her ability to swallow. With gastrostomy feeding she is expected to live for an additional 30 years or more. Her medical bills are the responsibility of the state of Missouri.

Ms. Cruzan's parents asked that the gastrostomy feedings be withdrawn, and sought a court order when the doctors and hospital refused to carry out their request. The trial judge granted their petition and authorized "the co-guardians to exercise [Ms. Cruzan's] constitutionally guaranteed liberty to request the withholding of nutrition and hydration" and instructed the co-guardians to exercise their legal authority consistent with her "best interests." The state and the guardian *ad litem* appealed.

Chief Justice Edward D. Robertson capsulized the Missouri Supreme Court's four-to-three opinion at the end of the first paragraph: "A single issue is presented: May a guardian order that all nutrition and hydration be withheld from an incompetent ward who is in a persistent vegetative state, who is neither dead . . . nor terminally ill? Because we find that the trial court erroneously declared the law, we reverse."[25]

It is difficult to discern just what basis the court had to reach this decision. It almost immediately noted, for example, that this is a "case of first impression" in Missouri, and cited more than 50 cases from 16 other states that have dealt with similar cases. It concluded that "nearly unanimously, those courts have found a way to allow persons wishing to die, or those who seek the death of a ward, to meet the end sought." This, of course, mistakes the question posed by these cases—almost none of the patients involved wished to die, and the guardians did not "seek" their deaths. Rather, the core issue was *the right to refuse treatment* that was unwanted or intolerable.

Because the court set *Cruzan* up as a "right to die" case rather than a "right to refuse treatment" case, it focused on irrelevant and misleading issues. For example, it focused on death and terminal illness without an apparent appreciation of the implications of either term. It used the phrase "Nancy is not dead" almost like a mantra in the opinion. Although the court seemed to see this as a major discovery, no one was arguing that the law could or should require guardians to provide artificial feeding to their deceased wards.

The court also stated repeatedly that the *Quinlan* case was irrelevant because Karen Quinlan was "terminally ill" even though the New Jersey Supreme Court *never* used the phrase to describe her. Karen Quinlan was in almost every way identical to Nancy Cruzan: a young woman in a persistent vegetative state who could live indefinitely with mechanical assistance, but who would never regain consciousness. Indeed, the only real difference between Ms. Quinlan and Ms. Cruzan is that while Ms. Quinlan was being maintained on both a mechanical ventilator and artificial feeding, Ms. Cruzan requires only the latter. But as the New

Jersey Supreme Court held in *Conroy*[26] and *Jobes*,[27] this is legally a meaningless distinction.

Although the Missouri court was very skeptical both about using the right of privacy as a basis for medical treatment decisions, and about treating artificial feeding as medical care, it ultimately did not reject either view. Instead it relied almost exclusively on the state's interest in preserving life (at least when continued care "does not cause pain" and is not particularly "burdensome to the patient," the patient "is not dead" nor "terminally ill," and cannot make a personal decision because of present incompetence). The court does not say, however, if or how these conclusions apply to antibiotics, CPR, or other medical interventions Ms. Cruzan might need to survive.

A recurring theme is the state's interest in life, regardless of its quality. If there is a holding in the *Cruzan* decision, it seems to be that the state can *never* take quality of life into consideration in acquiescing a decision to withdraw treatment from an incompetent individual, so long as the individual's life can be medically sustained without pain. But by protecting only Ms. Cruzan's interest in avoiding pain, the court ignores here interests in autonomy and personal dignity, and degrades and dehumanizes her.

Why have almost all other courts permitted patients or their surrogates to refuse treatment under similar circumstances? The reason is that those courts focused on the liberty interests of handicapped citizens, but the *Cruzan* court focused instead on laying the groundwork for a possible reversal of *Roe* v. *Wade*. The court, for example, expended great effort in criticizing the entire concept of the right of privacy. And in making its primary point on the state's unqualified interest in life, the court relied heavily not only on the state's new "Rights of the Terminally Ill Act," but also on its new abortion act (the one reviewed in *Webster*). As amended in 1986, its statement of purpose is:

> It is the intention of the . . . state of Missouri to grant the right to life to all humans, born and unborn, and to regulate abortion to the full extent permitted by the Constitution of the United States, decisions of the United States Supreme Court, and federal statutes.

The Act further defines "unborn child" as "the offspring of human beings from the moment of conception until birth," and viability as "when the life of the unborn child may be continued indefinitely outside the womb by natural or artificial *life-support systems*" [emphasis added by the court]. *Cruzan* is transformed into an abortion opinion. The court winds up by concluding simply that if life can be supported "indefinitely . . . by natural or artificial life-support systems," then it must be because of Missouri's unlimited interest in "the right to life of all humans."

The *Cruzan* case, now before the U.S. Supreme Court, is a hard case because we do not have clear evidence of Ms. Cruzan's wishes, because it is a feeding tube case, and because there is no evidence that Ms. Cruzan is suffering from the treatment. Nonetheless, any principled analysis would have to confront these issues directly, and focus ultimately on Ms. Cruzan herself and the decisions that must be made for her treatment.

Unfortunately, the Missouri Supreme Court made the case appear easy by treating Ms. Cruzan as a disembodied woman who cannot be hurt and who has no interests in either autonomy or dignity, but whose continued life is required by the state to uphold an abstract principle. In short, she is treated like a viable neonate, and Missouri's new antiabortion law is used to justify keeping her alive. The problem, of course, is that Ms. Cruzan has liberty and dignity interests that a newborn does not have, and the state's interests are permitted to overcome them only because her interests are ignored.

Nancy Cruzan lies in a hospital, her every bodily function being tended to by strangers; she will never regain consciousness; she indicated she would never want to survive like this, and her loving parents believe it would be in her best interests to have artificial feeding ended so that she can die in peace. If this request is not granted, she (and they) may have to continue to survive what is for them a living hell for 30 or more years so that four justices on the Missouri Supreme Court can say they "err on the side of life." The only solace in this opinion for Missouri citizens is that the court does seem to say that even though it views the right to refuse life-sustaining treatment as inalienable, competent adults do have this right and can exercise it prospectively provided they make their wishes known by clear and convincing evidence.

Patients who are permanently unconscious do present society with a major problem. But not the one identified by the court. There is ample precedent for following these patients' wishes regarding termination of treatment, if they are known. Like the trial court judge, I think there is sufficient evidence that Nancy herself would not want her life maintained this way, and her wishes should be honored.

Even if I did not so believe, however, and concluded that we could not know her own wishes, it seems to me that those courts that have permitted the next-of-kin (and/or the legal guardian) to make a determination consistent with their view of a patient's "best interests" are correct. If Ms. Cruzan's wishes are not sufficiently known, her parents (who are also her guardians) should be able to make the decision on her behalf as the people who know and love her best. Not to permit this deprives her of her family as well as her right to refuse treatment. It is true that permitting another to exercise choice on her behalf (since she is no longer capable of choosing anything) is not the same as permitting her to exercise choice. Nonetheless, unless we permit her family or guardian to make the choice for her, the doctors and hospital end up making it instead. The result is that the institution in which she resides gets to make her decisions, and that she can be forced to live for the sake of the state. This result should be seen as intolerable in a free society dedicated to preserving individual liberty and human dignity.[28]

COMBINING BIRTH AND DEATH: THE CASE OF ANGELA CARDER

The right to terminate a pregnancy and the right to refuse treatment came together in the case of a terminally ill, pregnant woman, Angela Carder, a 26-year-old married woman who had suffered from cancer since she was 13 years old.[29] About 25 weeks into her pregnancy, she was admitted to George Washington University Hospital, and a massive tumor was found in her lung. Physicians determined that she would die within a short time. Her husband, her mother, and her physicians agreed that keeping her comfortable while she died was what she wanted, and that her wishes should be honored. This was communicated to a hospital administrator, who called legal counsel, who in turn asked a judge to come to the hospital to decide what to do.

A District of Columbia Superior Court judge rushed to the hospital where he set up "court." After a hearing, the judge issued his opinion orally. The centerpiece was Ms. Carder's terminal condition. In the judge's words, "The uncontroverted medical testimony is that Angela will probably die within the next 24 to 48 hours." He did "not clearly know what Angela's present views are" respecting the cesarean section, but found that the fetus had a 50 to 60% chance to survive and less than a 20% chance for serious handicap. The judge concluded: "It's not an easy decision to make, but given the choices, the Court is of the view the fetus should be given the opportunity to live."

The court reconvened shortly thereafter when informed that Ms. Carder, who had been unconscious, was awake and communicating. The chief of obstetrics reported that she "clearly communicated" and "very clearly mouthed words several times, 'I don't want it done. I don't want it done. I don't want it done.'" Nonetheless, without even talking to Ms. Carder herself, the judge reaffirmed his original order. Less than an hour later, three judges heard a request for a stay, over the telephone, and denied it.

The cesarean section was performed, and the nonviable fetus died approximately 2 hours later. Ms. Carder, now confronted with both recovery from major surgery and the knowledge of her child's death, died approximately 2 days later. Five months later, the Court of Appeals issued its written opinion.[30] The opinion reads more like a Hallmark sympathy card than a judicial pronouncement. Its first paragraph, for example, ends with the following sentence: "Condolences are extended to those who lost the mother and child." The opinion is fatally flawed. The most serious error is the statement that "as a matter of law, the right of a woman to an abortion is different and distinct from her obligations to the fetus once she has decided not to timely terminate her pregnancy." This is incorrect as both a factual and a legal matter. Ms. Carder never "decided not to timely terminate her pregnancy," and because of her fetus' affect on her health, under *Roe* v. *Wade* she could have authorized her pregnancy to be terminated (to protect her health) at any time prior to her death. Moreover, had the roles been reversed, and an abortion was required to save Angela Carder's life, no legal principle would permit a judge to order the abortion against her will.

Another basis on which the opinion rests is that a parent cannot refuse treatment necessary to save the life of a child (true), and therefore a pregnant women cannot refuse treatment necessary to save the life of her fetus (false). The child must be treated because parents have obligations to act in the "best interests" of their children (as defined by child neglect laws), and treatment in no way compromises the bodily integrity of the parents. Fetuses, however, are not independent persons and cannot be treated without invading the mother's body. Treating the fetus against the will of the mother requires us to degrade and dehumanize the mother and treat her as an inert container. This *is* acceptable once the mother is dead, but it is never acceptable when the mother is alive. The court seems to understand this and thus ultimately justifies its opinion on the basis that Ms. Carder was as good as dead, and had no "good health" to be "sacrificed." "The cesarean section would not significantly affect Ms. Carder's condition because she had, at best, two days of sedated life."

But this reasoning will not do. It would, for example, permit the involuntary removal of vital organs prior to death when they were needed to "save a life." But if the child had already been born, no court would require its mother to undergo major surgery for its sake (for example, a kidney or partial liver "donation") no matter how dire the potential consequences of refusal to the child.

This unprincipled opinion was thankfully vacated by the full bench in early 1988[31] and thus has no legal value as precedent. But it dramatically illustrates the general rule that judges should never go to the hospital to make emergency treatment decisions. Rushed to an unfamiliar environment, asked to make a decision under great stress, and having no time either for reflection or for study of existing law and precedents, a judge cannot act judiciously. Facts cannot be properly developed, and the law cannot be accurately determined or fairly applied to the facts. The "emergency hearing" scenario is an invitation to arbitrariness and the exercise of raw force.

Unlike *Cruzan*, this was *not* a hard case. If there really were facts in dispute, a case conference involving the patient, family, and all attending health care personnel could have been held to assess them. Direct communication with the patient is almost always the most useful and constructive response to "problems" like those presented by this case. Calling a judge is usually a counterproductive, panic reaction; and decisions to "err on the side of life" can be deadly.

CONCLUSIONS

What can we conclude from all this? First, the abortion and refusing treatment cases illustrate that the criminal law is a blunt and often arbitrary instrument that takes little account of personal beliefs, individual dignity, or family wishes. It seems especially inappropriate in areas in which there are strong disagreements among major segments of society, and in which beliefs seem more a product of religious doctrine than moral reflection. Second, however denoted, the "right of privacy" offers protection from arbitrary governmental interference in matters involving conception, pregnancy, birth, and refusing treatment. The expansion of the right of privacy into the area of refusing life-sustaining treatment seems perfectly appropriate, since decisions about medical treatment and death are intensely personal ones that affect individuals profoundly, and almost never affect others or society at that level. Third, decisions about birth and death should generally be left to the individuals involved, because they are ultimately questions of profound moral values rather than proper subjects for the criminal law. None of the criminal laws goals—punishment, deterrence, and rehabilitation—have much applicability to decisions to terminate a pregnancy or a medical intervention. The criminal law, by bringing police, judges, and prosecutors into the picture, demeans pregnant women and dying patients by decreeing that they are not fit moral agents to make decisions about their own lives and their own futures.

This is not to argue that birth and death issues are unimportant. Rather it is to argue that the way we deal with them lies in the arena of the morality of aspiration, rather than in the arena of the morality of duty. As Lon Fuller has put it in the general context, "There is no way by which the law can compel a man to live up to the excellences of which he is capable."[32] In birth and death we can go further: the criminal law can only make extraordinarily difficult decisions seem black and white. But pretending dusk is either day or night ignores rather than confronts reality—the difficulty of personal responsibility for decisions at the beginning and end of life.

More than a decade ago, shortly after coming to the United States from Russia, novelist Alexander Solzhenitsyn was unflattering in his view of the United States as a culture dominated by law. He noted that while a society without any objective legal scale is "terrible, a society with no other scale but the legal one is not quite worthy of man either." As he accurately argued:

> A society that is based on the letter of the law and never reaches any higher is taking small advantage of the high level of human possibilities. The letter of the law is too cold and formal to have a beneficial influence on society. Whenever the tissue of life is woven of legalistic relations, there is an atmosphere of mediocrity, paralysing man's noblest impulses.[33]

Mediocrity and paralysis almost seem the norm in modern medicine as it characterizes itself with overconcern with legal liability and the practice of defensive medicine—medicine done for the benefit of the physician rather than the patient. Criminalizing conduct by patients that physicians and/or society disapprove of will lead only to further paralysis and mediocrity. The road to a higher moral plane is not through the criminal courtrooms of America, but by a renewed emphasis on reflection and personal responsibility.

We do need a rededication to responsible sexual relations, responsible pregnancy, and responsible parenthood. We do need to deal with the reality of our mortality and come to conclusions about our medical care at the end of life, leaving directions in the form of living wills and durable powers of attorney for our loved ones to follow. We do need to assure universal access to adequate medical care. But we do not need more laws to restrict the activities of pregnant women, to require women to continue pregnancies against their will, to force individuals to be subjected to medical treatment against their will, or to require families to stand helplessly by while their children are maintained like plants in permanent comas for the sake of the state. If the U.S. Supreme Court gives Congress and the states the legal authority to restrict abortion rights and force treatment, let us join the legislative battle to reject the invitation to turn matters of personal morality into matters of society's criminal law.

ADDENDUM

Since this chapter was written, The United States Supreme Court has affirmed the *Cruzan* decision by a vote of 5 to 4 (June 1990); and the District of Columbia Court of Appeals has vacated the lower court opinion in *A.C.* [Angela Carder-Ed.] and issued a lengthy written opinion concluding that "in virtually all cases" (including *A.C.*) the decision of the pregnant woman must control (7 to 1; April 1990).

NOTES AND REFERENCES

1. *Webster* v. *Reproductive Health Services*, 109 S. Ct. 3040 (1989).
2. L. Greenhouse, "High Court Facing Fight on Abortion, Privacy and Death," *The New York Times*, Oct. 2, 1989, p. 1.
3. N. Brozan, "O'Connor Proposes Order of Nuns to Fight Abortion and Euthanasia," *The New York Times*, Nov. 4, 1989, p. 31.
4. G. Williams, *The Sanctity of Life and the Criminal Law* (New York: Knopf, 1966), x.
5. L. Fuller, *The Morality of Law,* rev. ed. (New Haven: Yale University Press, 1964), 5–6.
6. *Buck* v. *Bell*, 274 U.S. 200 (1927).
7. *Skinner* v. *Oklahoma*, 316 U.S. 535 (1942) [emphasis added].
8. *In the Matter of Grady*, 85 N.J. 235, 426 A.2d 467 (1981).
9. *Griswold* v. *Connecticut*, 381 U.S. 479 (1965).
10. *Eisenstadt* v. *Baird*, 405 U.S. 438 (1972).
11. A consistent majority believes that abortion is immoral in most cases. Nonetheless, overwhelming majorities believe that abortions should be available in cases of rape, incest, and severe genetic abnormality, and more than two-thirds consistently say that although they believe abortion to be wrong or immoral, the ultimate decision should be made by a woman and her physician rather than by government decree. M. A. Lamanna, "Social Sciences and Ethical Issues: The Policy Implications of Poll Data on Abortion," in *Abortion: Understanding Differences,* Daniel and Sidney Callahan, eds. (New York: Plenum Press, 1984), 1–23; and E. J. Dionne, Jr., "Poll Finds Ambivalence on Abortion Persists in U.S.," *The New York Times*, Aug. 3, 1989, p. A18.
12. *Roe* v. *Wade*, 410 U.S. 113 (1973).
13. R. Woodward and S. Armstrong, *The Brethren: The Inside Story of the Supreme Court* (New York: Simon and Schuster, 1979).
14. G. J. Annas, "The Supreme Court, Privacy and Abortion," *New England Journal of Medicine*, 321 (1989): 1200–1203.
15. N. D. Hunter, "Time Limits on Abortion," in *Reproductive Laws for the 1990's,* S. Cohen and N. Taub, eds. (Clifton, N.J.: Humana Press, 1989), 129–153.
16. *Harris* v. *McRae*, 448 U.S. 297 (1980).

17. S. Elias and G. J. Annas, *Reproductive Genetics and the Law* (Chicago: Yearbook Medical Publishers, 1987), 143–162.

18. L. H. Glantz, "Abortion: A Decade of Decisions," in *Genetics and the Law III*, A. Milunsky and G. J. Annas, eds. (New York: Plenum Press, 1985), 295–307.

19. *Supra*, note 1.

20. Brief of the American Medical Association *et al.* in Support of Appellees, No. 88–605 (1989).

21. *Akron* v. *Center for Reproductive Health*, 462 U.S. 416 (1983) (O'Connor, dissenting).

22. *In the Matter of Quinlan*, 355 A. 2d 647 (N.J. 1976).

23. *JFK Memorial Hospital* v. *Heston*, 279 A.2d 670 (N.J. 1971).

24. *Superintendent of Belchertown* v. *Saikewicz*, 370 N.E. 2d 417 (MA. 1977).

25. *Cruzan* v. *Harmon*, 110 S.Ct. 2d 284 (MO. 1990).

26. *In the Matter of Claire Conroy*, 486 A.2d 1209 (N.J. 1985).

27. *In the Matter of Jobes*, 529 A.2d 437 (N.J. 1987).

28. The material on *Cruzan* has been adapted from G. J. Annas, "The Insane Root Takes Reason Prisoner," *Hastings Center Report*, 19, 1 (1989): 29–31.

29. The facts of this case are taken from the transcript of the hearing. See also G. J. Annas, "She's Going to Die: The Case of Angela C," *Hastings Center Report*, 18, 1 (1988): 23–25, and G. J. Annas, *The Rights of Patients* (Carbondale, IL: Southern Illinois University Press, 1989), 128–130.

30. *In the Matter of A.C.* [Angela Carder-Ed.], 533 A.2d 611 (App. D.C. 1987).

31. *In the Matter of A.C.*, 539 A.2d 203 (App. D.C. 1988).

32. Fuller, p. 9, n. 5.

33. Aleksandr I. Solzhenitsyn, "The Exhausted West," *Harvard Magazine* (July/August 1978): 22.

II
RETHINKING CONTROVERSIAL QUESTIONS

3

Abortion in a Pluralistic Society: Can Freedom and Moral Probity Coexist?

Daniel Callahan

At the heart of much moral debate in America lies a simple and popular conviction: the law should leave to the individual conscience choice about those acts that are private, do not command a moral consensus, and are not harmful to others. I will call this the pluralistic proposition. The abortion debate of the past three decades has, in great part, been about this proposition. Those who call themselves "pro-choice" argue that the abortion choice is private and personal to women and should thus be left to them without the interference of the law. The "pro-life" side, by contrast, has held that the decisive harm abortion does to the fetus and its right to life removes it from the private realm and makes it a matter of legitimate government regulation.

I do not want here to examine directly the struggle between those two positions, the general structure of which is by now all too painfully familiar from the endless public debate. I want instead to look at the subject of abortion as a case study of the problems and paradoxes of the pluralistic proposition, particularly as it has manifested itself in the logic and politics of the pro-choice position. One question, above all, troubles me. Is it possible, simultaneously and with equal seriousness, to hold that abortion should (1) be left to the individual and private choice of women, and (2) that each such decision should be understood as a genuine moral choice, one that can be good or bad, right or wrong?

This question is important for the abortion debate, but no less important for many other ethical debates that come down to deciding between private choice and government intervention. If we opt for private choice, what is this likely to mean to the idea of personal morality, and what are its possible social implications? Can we entertain a meaningful and substantive notion of personal morality in a pluralistic society? Or is it the case that the pluralistic proposition—in practice if not necessarily in theoretical formulation—encourages a thin and minimalistic, relativistic idea of personal morality? Could it be that a strong notion of pluralism requires a weak notion of personal morality, or that a strong notion of personal morality requires a weak notion of pluralism?

Why am I interested in these questions? Twenty-one years ago I published a book on abortion, *Abortion: Law, Choice and Morality*.[1] Reversing my own earlier convictions, I concluded that the universality of a resort to abortion even if illegal and dangerous, the inherently uncertain moral status of the fetus (at least the relatively early fetus), and the value in a pluralistic society of keeping the law out of controverted and delicate moral issues whenever possible made the "pro-choice" position morally and politically compelling. I have not changed my view on the legal issue in any significant way.

I also argued, no less strongly, that even though the choice should be the woman's, and that it should be a private choice, it was still a serious moral choice. Once women had the choice, it would then become important for them in their private lives to give thought to what would count as a morally justifiable choice; and it would be no less appropriate to have some public discussion about the standards and criteria appropriate for such choices, much as we might about other moral matters not subject to law but of common interest and importance. To be sure, the private moral wrestling would and could be a source of anguish and pain, but that is true of all critical moral choices, hardly unique to abortion. The goal that I proposed seemed, then, perfectly compatible with what I understand the pluralistic proposition to be: leave the choice to women but understand the choice to be a grave one, worthy of public no less than private reflection.

I could not have been more naive, more hopelessly optimistic, in thinking that such reflection would be acceptable. The pro-choice movement has in fact never known quite what to do with the moral issue. For most of its leaders, it is simply set aside altogether, left to the opaque sphere of personal morality, itself a subject of uncertainty and discomfort. Is it not the nature of personal morality, many seem to think, that it is so unique and idiosyncratic to the individual, so subject to private, self-determined moral standards, that nothing meaningful can be said about it, and certainly not enough for public debate? The tacit answer to this question is clear enough. There is a great deal of sociological literature on why women have abortions, and many interesting journalistic accounts of women's experience in making abortion decisions. Yet there is remarkably little written about how women *ought* to make such private decisions, that is, thoughtful writing on the appropriate moral uses of free choice for those who have the legal right to do so.

Yet if silence or uneasiness is the predominant response to the moral problem, there are others in the pro-choice movement—a small but seemingly growing minority—for whom even the idea of a discussion of the moral choice is repugnant.[2] They either want to declare that abortion is not, in its substance, a moral question at all (only the woman's *right* to choose an abortion is taken to be a moral issue), or that women should not have to struggle and suffer over the choice even if it is, or that, in any case, to concede that it is a *serious* moral choice and to have a public discussion about that choice is politically hazardous, the opening wedge of a discussion that could easily lead once again to a restriction of a woman's right to an abortion. Better to declare the whole topic of the morality of abortion off limits.

One way or another, then, the pro-choice movement has not been able to tolerate the fullness of the pluralistic proposition. It can support the choice side more readily than the morality side. At best it is uneasy about the moral issue, at worst dismissive and hostile toward it.

That stance has an important practical implication for the future of the pro-choice movement: its inability or unwillingness to come to grips with the moral issue threatens its political credibility. The majority of Americans, the public opinion polls indicate, are greatly troubled about the moral reasons for abortion in different circumstances.[3] Not all private reasons are accepted as equally valid, and a large proportion of people report themselves uncertain about their own views, not just those of others. The pro-life movement has effectively capitalized on this uncertainty, appealing to the moral uneasiness of many and bringing to the surface qualms and doubts shunted aside by the pro-choice movement.

If, for some people, to have choice is itself the beginning and end of morality, for most people it is just the beginning. It does not end until a supportable, justifiable choice has been made, one that can be judged right or wrong by the individual herself based on some reasonably serious, not patently self-interested way of thinking about ethics. That standard—central to every major ethical system and tradition—applies to the moral life generally, whether it be a matter of abortion or any other grave matter. An unwillingness to come to grips with that standard not only puts the pro-choice movement in jeopardy as a political force, it has a still more deleterious effect: it is a basic threat to moral honesty and integrity. The cost of failing to take seriously the personal moral issues is to court self-deception and to be drawn to employ arguments of expediency and evasion. I want to show how that has happened in at least some strands of the pro-choice movement and why it reduces the moral strength of that position.

Before I develop that thesis, however, a caution is in order. Despite the harsh things I have to say about elements of the pro-choice position, I think in the end it is the only one that is viable in our society. For all of its faults, it is the position I embrace. Though there is room for change and compromise, it would be a great loss to have the substance of *Roe* v. *Wade* overturned, that of leaving early abortions in the private hands of women and their physicians. I am searching for two things simultaneously: a *permanent* and *secure* place in American law for the right of women to make their own choice, and a far richer, more sensitive notion of the nature of that choice than is now commonly the case.

Let me begin that task by looking, first, at the history of arguments used by the pro-choice movement, that movement which in the 1973 *Roe* v. *Wade* decision achieved its greatest victory and which is now in jeopardy; and then, second, at the developments in the arguments since that time.

During the 1950s and into the late 1960s, the movement to legalize abortion rested on a number of contentions: that a vast number of illegal abortions was doing great harm to the health of women, killing and maiming them; that women should have available a backup to ineffective contraception, though the latter should always remain the primary method of birth control; that the number of unwanted pregnancies, thought to be large, should be reduced and only wanted children should be born—the welfare of children was as much at stake as that of women; that, while an abortion decision is and must be difficult morally and psychologically, a woman should have a right to make such a decision; and that, while abortion should be legally available and financially affordable, everything possible should be done to change those economic and domestic circumstances that force women into unwanted pregnancies.

Although this set of arguments looked strongly to the freedom and welfare of women, it was not exclusively a feminist argument by any means. It stressed the common benefits of abortion reform, particularly to children and the society, and it drew heavily on the pluralistic proposition, which bears on a wide range of personal choices for men and women, not simply the abortion choice for women.

Many of those arguments are still, of course, part of the movement. But there have been a number of developments since the early 1970s— some political, some scientific, and some ideological. The most obvious political change has been the emergence of a strong, well-organized and well-financed pro-life movement. It has been able to press its case effectively in legislatures and with the general public (even though, remarkably, public opinion has remained remarkably stable and stationary on abortion for nearly two decades). Although this movement has often been stereotyped by its opponents as nothing but religious conservatism, that is hardly accurate. It has grass root support among many who are otherwise politically liberal. It has also of late gained the support of many women who are feminists. They see in abortion a resort to violence similar to that used for centuries by men against women: the use of power by the strong against the weak, both the physical power of violence and the cultural power to define the unwanted out of the human community altogether.[4] More generally, the pro-life movement has found its greatest strength in its focus on precisely that issue that the pro-choice movement has found most discomforting and awkward: the moral status of the fetus.

The most important scientific developments have been threefold. There is the growing medical interest in fetal health and development, a trend that has nothing directly to do with the abortion issue, but reflecting research and public health concerns. There is the lowering age of fetal viability, now down to 24 weeks, a result of the great improvements in neonatology (though perhaps, for the time being, stalled at that level). There is the widespread use of the sonogram, allowing a woman to see her fetus *in utero*.[5] Taken together, these scientific developments have brought the fetus more squarely before the public eye. The pro-life movement did not create that trend, but has effectively capitalized on it by tying it into its moral focus on the fetus.

The most striking ideological development has been the emergence into leadership positions in the pro-choice movement of some feminists who have scanted many of the original arguments for abortion reform. They have shifted the emphasis almost entirely to a woman's right to an abortion, whatever her reasons and whatever the consequences. Much less is heard about the social harm of unwanted pregnancies, much less about the terrible or tragic choice posed by an abortion, much less about the moral nature of the choice, and practically nothing about the need to reduce the number of abortions, now running at a rate of 1.6 million a year. No number of abortions seems to be too many.

It is as if, in face of the pro-life movement, some feminist leaders have decided to be as single-minded and unmeasured as their opponents; and they have become in many respects a mirror-image of them. If the pro-life movement exclusively stresses the rights of the fetus, then the pro-choice movement must exclusively stress the rights of women. If the pro-life movement says that abortion is oppressive and murderous, the pro-choice movement must then say it is liberating and morally unimportant. If the pro-life movement says that every abortion choice is wrong, whatever the reason, then the pro-choice leadership implies that every choice is right, whatever the choice. From a movement that in the 1950 and 1960s was measured, careful, and open to larger concerns, it now runs the risk of becoming narrow and ideologically rigid. I do not claim that this characterization is true of all pro-choice leaders—far from it—only that it is strongly present, and growing, and in a way that was not the case two decades ago. It has come to overshadow the writings and work of other feminists, no less intent on preserving women's freedom of choice, but also on setting that freedom in a context of the common good of men and women, children, and families.

Why has this shift taken place? The most obvious reasons are the growing pressures and successes of the pro-life movement, forcing a more defensive, intransigent position; the prospect of a Supreme Court gutting or reversal of *Roe* v. *Wade;* and the impact of the media, with its predilection for polarized positions, encouraging one-dimensionality on both sides of the debate. Yet we might speculate on a more subtle additional possibility: that of the actual difficulty of managing the pluralistic proposition in the face of insistent moral issues that cannot be successfully denatured by exclusive reduction to choice.

Public opinion polls over the years have persistently displayed two distinctive features. When asked a *general* question about the right of women to have an abortion, a majority favor such a right; it has been steadily supportive of *Roe* v. *Wade*. At the same time, when questioned more precisely, a majority also want morally to distinguish among abortion choices. In that respect, the public has never been unambiguously pro-choice or pro-life; some 60% of the public falls in a zone of ambivalence and nuance.[6]

The pro-choice movement is unable to respond effectively to these findings, partly because of its own ideology (which wants no such distinctions) and partly because of deficiencies in the pluralistic proposition on which it relies to make its general case. The consequence of these deficiencies is that, when pressed on the personal moral issues, the pro-choice leadership usually reacts with anger, confusion, or denial. It does not know what else to do with them.

Why has this happened? I offer a hypothesis. To make its advocacy case, the pro-choice movement has partially relied on a set of beliefs and assertions that are either false or highly misleading. It has had to do that because, if looked at too closely, the actual complexity of the abortion situation raises disturbing questions about both the political realities and issues of personal morality. To admit that complexity would be to admit the importance of some portions of the pro-life argument, a highly distressing prospect. I offer a partial list of those assertions, counterpoised against what I take to be the more complex truth of the matter.

1. *Abortion restrictions represent a war of men against women, with men intent on keeping women in reproductive thralldom.* Yet every survey for nearly 20 years shows women themselves divided on the issue, marginally but consistently more opposed to fully permissive abortion than men. The strongest supporters of legal abortion over the years have been young males. Should we be surprised at that? Molly Yard, President of NOW, said after the *Webster* decision that the Court has begun "a war against women." The polls would suggest that abortion is as much a war among women as against women (with class and education a significant element of that war). Faye D. Ginsburg's important recent book, *Contested Lives,* underscores that point.[7]

2. *Abortion should not be promoted as a primary means of birth control, but as a backup to a contraceptive failure.* Yet some 40% of all abortions are now repeat abortions, a figure that has steadily grown over the years. There are, moreover, some 1.6 million abortions a year, with no diminution in sight. Those figures suggest, though do not prove, a primary and growing dependence for many on abortion as the first line of defense against unwanted pregnancy, not a backup method (and reminiscent of the pattern that developed in Eastern Europe in the aftermath of abortion liberalization in the 1960s and 1970s).

3. *Abortion will diminish the dependence of women on men, giving them full control over their reproduction.* If legal abortion has given women more choice, it has also given men more choice as well. They now have a potent new weapon in the old business of manipulating and abandoning women. For if women can have abortions, then there is no compelling leverage for women to use in demanding that men take responsibility for the children they procreate. That men have long coerced women into abortion when it suits their purposes is well known but rarely mentioned. Data reported by the Alan Guttmacher Institute indicate that some 30% of women have an abortion because someone else, not the woman, wants it.[8] The same data indicate that is not necessarily the exclusive reason, but it is remarkably difficult to find much pro-choice probing into the reality of coerced abortions. It is as if there is an embarrassed, sheepish silence on what would seem a matter of obvious concern for those committed to choice.

4. *Given freedom of choice, women will make free choices.* Why is it, then, that many women feel coerced economically into having an abortion? (Poor black women, mainly young, are proportionately the largest group to choose abortion.) Why is it, then, that there is now a whole genre of literature and reports of women who regret their abortions, who felt coerced by others or their social circumstances into having an abortion they would not otherwise have chosen?[9] Although it may be an accident

that resources for the poor have diminished in parallel with the increased access to abortion, exactly that has happened. But is it wholly an accident that our country combines the world's most liberal abortion laws with the poorest social support and systems for women, mothers and children?[10]

5. *It does not matter what choice women make as long as they have the freedom to make their own choice.* But that is a hard position to sustain, even for the single-minded, when the choice is to abort a female fetus simply because it is female, or to have an abortion to please (or spite) a husband or boy friend, or to have a repeat abortion because of a casual attitude toward the use of contraceptives, or to conceive fetuses for experimental purposes or commercial profit.

I cite that list of arguments to show that "choice" covers a multitude of realities, not all of them quite so tidy as some mainline pro-choice ideology would have it. Those realities reveal a disturbingly obvious point: not all opponents of abortion are men, not all arguments against abortion are antiwoman, and not each and every abortion choice is equally justifiable, either because of the social circumstances or setting of the choice, or because of the actual content of the choice.

Of course to concede even the moral possibility that some abortion choices could be reprehensible, to admit that some choices can be morally wrong, would be to agree that choice itself is not the end of the moral matter. As a theoretical issue, the pluralistic proposition surely encompasses that possibility. To admit that much in the case of particular abortion choices, however, would be to show the hazards of the pluralistic proposition in its actual political usage. At the very least, it would be to concede implicitly that the fetus has enough moral status to force a judgment that not all reasons for its destruction are morally defensible. There are good choices, and there are bad choices.

Even contemplating this possibility poses a hard dilemma for the pro-choice leadership. Consider two possible alternatives here. One of them is to reject altogether the contention that abortion represents a moral choice of any consequence, and some take that route. But that view is hardly likely to be persuasive to most pro-choice supporters, who know better. The other alternative is to concede the validity of the moral worries, the importance of the moral substance of choice, and thereby open the door to a public moral discussion of abortion itself. That would require seriously considering at least some pro-life arguments and perspectives, and would of course lay the basis for a moral rejection of some abortions, perhaps many.

Note an interesting parallel. A number of prominent feminists—including Betty Friedan and Gloria Steinem, it might be recalled—came to reject a pure choice ideology in the case of surrogate motherhood (during the debate over the Baby M case). The choice of becoming a surrogate mother, they argued, is not necessarily a good choice or beneficial to women, however much it may have the virtue of being a choice that a woman can legally make. That was a little-noted revolution in feminist thinking, though it was foreshadowed by those feminists who have condemned pornography and prostitution even in cases where women freely choose to take part. The same kind of thinking applied to the abortion debate would represent a genuine upheaval—asking not just whether it is good for women to have choice, but to ask also what constitutes a good choice. How can it make sense to favor the right to choice, but to be morally indifferent about the use of that right? We all favor the right to free speech, but we are not unconcerned—nor do we withhold our public condemnation—when that right is used to insult or demean those of other races. Those are not thought to be, nor are they, contradictory positions.

I conclude that only the second alternative noted above is tenable: to admit the moral seriousness of the abortion choice. I have already suggested one set of reasons for moving in that direction: the high price paid in credibility for evasion of problems of real moral concern to probably a majority of pro-choice supporters (and surely a great concern to those who are not certain just where they stand). Such a move will surely be risky. Once they start taking the moral choice seriously, some people are likely to change their position on abortion in general. Yet in the long run, if the pro-choice position is to prevail, it will have to run such risks. It has not so far planted solid roots, and it has, out of anxiety and muddle, put to one side moral questions that are as urgent as they are real. More generally, the pluralistic proposition cannot itself well endure unless it finds a stronger place for a consideration of private moral choices. A strong commitment to legal freedom and choice combined with a weak commitment to substantive moral examination and ethical choice is an unsatisfactory combination. The latter simply goes underground, eating away corrosively at the commitment to legal freedom.

Is it possible in the case of abortion to combine legal freedom and seriousness about the moral questions? That would require the meeting of at least four conditions: (1) recognizing that the pro-choice position represents only one important moral tradition in our culture, and must exist in tension with and appreciation of the no less important tradition embodied in the pro-life movement, that of a respect for life; (2) accepting the need for active public debate about individual moral choices and the likelihood that some will be judged more negatively than others; (3) accepting the necessity for some compromise in the law as a way of taking seriously the objections of the pro-life position; and (4) agreeing on the need to make every effort to change those economic and social circumstances that lead women to make coerced abortion choices, and on the need for meaningful counseling of women who are considering abortion.

1. *Abortion and the Traditions of Morality.* One reason for the intensity and intractability of the abortion debate is that it pits two important moral traditions against each other: that of respect for choice, and that of respect for life. The pro-life position speaks eloquently and meaningfully about the value of nascent, defenseless life. It is a morally serious position, one compatible with a wide range of other values that seek to protect and preserve life.

Where it fails, in the eyes of many of us, however, is in moving from its premise of respect for life to its conclusion that embryonic or fetal life merits the same protection as life after birth. At the least, that is a difficult question, not so perspicuously self-evident as pro-life advocates would have us believe.

A pro-life position that would resolutely put to one side the value of free choice in grappling with, and acting on, that question must fail to make a fully persuasive case. It assumes that it has solved a moral problem for everyone that has, in actuality, never found any single and enduring historical solution. It confuses moral fervor and noble intentions with ethical justification. It would impose on the unwilling a position that does not command their moral agreement and would force them to act against their conscience.

To say all that is not to imply that the pro-choice position is free of problems. There are, in fact, varied ways of formulating that position, and it makes a difference which one chooses. A pro-choice position that would make the value of early human life depend solely on private choice and the individual exercise of power—the view that a woman confers value on a fetus by her decision to accept it—fails to understand the importance of communal safeguards against capricious power over life and death. It is no less insensitive to the all-too-common tendency to define out of the human community those lives that are threatening or burdensome. It is prone morally to confuse being unwanted with being valueless, a blurring of categories that puts the value of all human life at risk. A viable pro-choice stance for the future must come to grips with those hazards in far more effective ways than it has done in the past. The first step is to be willing to talk about them, having the nerve to put aside worries about the political hazards of doing so.

It *is* hazardous. But the importance of running that risk is that by doing so, the pro-choice movement will put itself in a far more secure long-term position. The state of public opinion provides one reason for thinking about this possibility. Why is there, as public opinion polls suggest, a broad agreement on the general right of women to make an abortion choice, yet considerable disagreement on morally acceptable reasons for abortion? The most plausible reason is that most people are trying to find a suitable balance between the traditions of choice and those of respect for life. Although *Roe* v. *Wade* is tolerable for a majority if asked a yes or no question, it does not capture well the shadings of their actual feelings and evaluation; it is too crude. In the long run, a nuanced position that makes some distinctions among and between reasons for abortion is likely to be taken more seriously than one that wants, once and for all, to resolve the tension. A pro-choice position that opposes any political compromise fails to understand that, for most people, their own moral judgment is already a compromise.

2. *Moral Choice and Moral Judgment.* Only a willingness to make room for an ongoing—and no doubt never-ending—debate about the morality of individual abortion choices can preserve the status of abortion as a serious moral issue. A pro-choice movement unwilling or unable to do that will be forever in jeopardy, hiding from itself but not from others its underlying moral insecurity. In practice that kind of openness will mean accepting the likelihood that some reasons for abortion will be judged reasonable and acceptable, and others unreasonable and unacceptable. It no less means that women will and should have a difficult and highly troubling debate with themselves about their own abortions and will, if the public discussion has been full and rich, have to struggle with the conflicting moral views. Nothing has so baffled me over the years as the faintly patronizing, paternalistic way in which, in the name of choice, it has been thought necessary to protect women from serious moral struggle.

I take it to be a good rule of ethical thinking that an important moral choice is one that can give a principled defense of itself and that is not, under most circumstances, simply a self-interested defense of personal preference (called ethical egoism in the philosophical literature). In this case, that would, at least, require some sensitive reflection of the values encompassed in that moral tradition that presses for a respect for life. It should not, moreover, be assumed that, just because there is psychological anguish or ambivalence about abortion, there is moral seriousness present; they are not necessarily the same. Anguish and ambivalence can result from trying to decide what one really wants to do, fear of the procedure itself, worry about the reaction of others. Serious ethical reflection goes beyond those matters. It requires thinking carefully about the moral status of the fetus, and about the best way to live a life and to shape a set of moral values and ideals.

3. *Compromise and Accommodation.* The Supreme Court, in its 1989 *Webster* decision, gave to the states the right to set some conditions on

abortion, and it will probably allow even further restrictions in the future. It may even overturn the *Roe* v. *Wade* decision, but that is thought less likely. An immediate response of the pro-choice leadership to *Webster* was hostility to the decision and to any and all compromise. Planned Parenthood, in a series of advertisements after the decision, said that there could be "no middle ground." That kind of stance is a mistake. The *Webster* decision already assures that there will be such ground, like it or not. More importantly, it seems increasingly clear that, *with some compromise*, an accommodation might be developed that would have a good chance of both enduring and allowing for the great majority of present abortions.

What accommodations might be reasonable? A restriction on late abortions, already made more difficult by the *Webster* decision, would meet widespread approval. A large number of hospitals have, for some years, established an informal cutoff point of 20 weeks, so a restriction of this kind would not have a major impact. A parental notification requirement for minors seeking abortion would win widespread support as well (even if, I believe, it would have some unhappy, damaging results). A continuing limitation on the use of federal facilities, while also troublesome, is doubtless likely in the future. Most abortions are not carried out for strictly medical or health reasons, but for private and personal reasons. It is hard, then, to see how a strong case can be made for the use of federal or federally supported facilities in the face of widespread public opposition, and in the light of the pro-choice definition of abortion as a private matter, outside the scope of government intervention.

I do not claim that such compromises will be without pain. A number of women might in the future be denied abortions, for economic or other reasons, that are now available. I am only saying that compromises of this sort are most likely to find a middle ground that will be acceptable to public opinion, to be sustainable by the legislatures and courts, and yet also to be most likely to ensure that women will still be left with a wide range of choice in the future.

4. *Taking Choice Seriously.* There are three major obstacles to taking choice seriously. The first I have already discussed at length: the fear of, and reluctance to, even discuss openly what might count as an unjustifiable moral choice. The morality of the choice is thereby trivialized. The second obstacle is the absence of serious counseling on abortion, particularly in the clinics that do such a large number of abortions. Counselors rarely explore with women their own thinking, the implications for womens' lives of their choice, or the possibility that women are being influenced or coerced into abortions they would not otherwise want. There can be no serious choice apart from those conditions. If one

believes in real choice—in abortion or any other serious matter that requires reflection and psychological freedom—then the proposal in many states that there be a mandatory waiting period of a few days seems a reasonable accommodation for the pro-choice movement to make. A flat rejection of that possibility suggests a desire to maximize abortion rather than to increase choice.

I should stress that unless good counseling services were in place, I would be considerably less assured about going in this direction. There will, to be sure, be practical problems here. Good counseling programs are never easy to organize. But then the present situation is hardly adequate either. It allows women little occasion for considered and assisted reflection and inadequate help in implementing a range of different choices. This is even more true of the poor than the affluent.

Counseling will, however, have little meaning unless there is an enormous improvement in the services and social benefits available to women. The United States lags far beyond every other industrialized nation in the provision of protections, choices, and benefits for pregnant women and mothers. If abortion provides for some women a meaningful alternative to the bearing of a child they cannot afford and will be unable to care for properly, it also has the ironic effect of taking pressure off the government and society to give them decent help, which would allow them to choose instead to have the child. Abortion is often a cheap solution to deep social problems, and all the more seductive if it is dressed up in the language of choice, pretending that poor women really have meaningful choices. The only plausible way to resist that outcome is to make clear that abortion should never be an alternative to full and decent social policy, and that the presence of permissive abortion laws provides no excuse to avoid putting needed policy reforms into place.

What might an abortion policy in the future look like with that aim in mind and in light of the accommodations I have suggested? It would encompass two major ingredients. On the one hand, there would be a sharp restriction of late abortions, parental notification with teenagers, federally supported abortions only for medical or clear health reasons, mandatory counseling and waiting periods, and serious efforts to reduce the number of abortions, especially repeat abortions. There would be, on the other hand, a significant improvement in maternal and child benefits, improved counseling, and more effective family planning and contraceptive education and services.

The pro-choice movement would, in its future work, stress the need for serious choice, the moral character of that choice, and be receptive to public debate about standards for the making of private choice. Even if it comes to a different conclusion about the moral status of the fetus—as it doubtless will—the pro-choice side should show itself no less probing about the importance of that question than the pro-life side. That kind of probing will probably lead to a loss of some people from its side, perhaps many. But its willingness to engage in such probing, and to run that risk, will itself have a powerful appeal to many pro-life adherents who are themselves ambivalent about denying all choice to women. Some of them will come over.

If the pro-choice movement presents itself as principally a movement about the rights of women, it is likely to lose in the long run. The abortion issue is broader, deeper, and more complex than that. It is surely about those rights, but it is also about the welfare of families and children, about the obligations of males toward women and toward the children they procreate, and about the family and the place of childbearing within it. The pro-choice movement can show itself to be one of nuance and responsibility, of choice and moral seriousness, of women's right to self-determination and their demonstrated and undoubted capacity to put that commitment in the larger context of a common social good.

At stake here as well is the future of the pluralistic proposition. A pluralism that tries to buy social peace at the expense of moral probity, or considers public issues of far greater importance than private moral issues, cannot long endure. It will be beset from within by those who give thought to their private choices and who wonder about the meaning and impact of those choices in their lives and the lives of others. It will and should be troubled when it recognizes that many so-called private choices are shaped, even determined, by social circumstances and mores. The idea that we can draw a sharp line between the public and the private sphere, between public and private choices, is a great myth. They constantly influence and reflect each other.

A strong pluralism is one that just as actively debates the nature and content of private choice as it does that of public legal and political choice. The only crucial difference is this: its supporters agree that, however the debate about that content goes, it will and should in the end leave choice to the individual. The great weakness of the pro-life movement is that it has not been willing to trust individuals with free and private moral choice. The pro-choice movement has fallen into a different trap. It has been unwilling to trust the moral issues to public debate.

I hope that the pro-choice movement would now be willing to run that greatest of all risks (but the only one that seems to me credible for the common good): the willingness to entertain a robust, thick, and probing conception of personal morality, one that is just as strong in its way as the pluralism and toleration at the level of law and politics is in its way.

The pro-choice movement has tried to make do with a thin, near-to-vanishing idea of personal morality. That serves neither its own long-term interests nor those of the pluralistic proposition.

NOTES AND REFERENCES

1. Daniel Callahan, *Abortion: Law, Choice and Morality* (New York: Macmillan, 1970).

2. Jason DeParle, "Beyond the Legal Right: Why Liberals and Feminists Don't Like to Talk About the Morality of Abortion," *The Washington Monthly* (April 1989): 28–44.

3. E. J. Dionne, Jr., "Polls Find Ambivalence on Abortion Persists in U.S.," *The New York Times*, Aug. 3, 1989, p. A18.

4. Sidney Callahan, "Abortion and the Sexual Agenda," *Commonweal*, April 25, 1986: 232–238.

5. Daniel Callahan, "How Technology Is Reframing the Abortion Debate," *Hastings Center Report*, 16, 1 (February 1986): 33–42.

6. See Dionne, *ibid.*, and also *Gallup Poll Monthly* (April 1, 1990): 41.

7. Faye D. Ginsburg, *Contested Lives: The Abortion Debate in an American Community* (Berkeley: University of California Press, 1989).

8. Rachel Benson Gold, *Abortion and Women's Health* (New York: The Alan Guttmacher Institute, 1990), 20.

9. See, for instance, David C. Reardon, *Aborted Women: Silent No More* (Chicago: Loyola University Press, 1987).

10. Mary Ann Glendon, *Abortion and Divorce in American Law: American Failures and European Challenges* (Cambridge: Harvard University Press, 1987).

4

Morality and Choice: A Response to Daniel Callahan

Mark Washofsky

Any adequate response to Daniel Callahan's penetrating critique of the contemporary movement for abortion rights must begin with the admission that surely he is right. He is right when he reminds us that the availability of abortion does not imply that all abortions are morally justifiable. And he is probably right when he suggests that a morally "nuanced" position, one that distinguishes among good and bad reasons for abortion, stands a better chance of winning general acceptance than does an extremist view that does not seek, as he puts it, "a suitable balance between the traditions of choice and respect for life." (p. 67) He confronts the advocate of abortion rights with this challenge: Does the doctrine of choice have a foundation in morality? If "pro-choice" is based on nothing more substantial than what he calls the "pluralistic proposition," then the answer is surely no. An ideology that advocates the right of privacy and freedom of choice for "consenting adults" while it pays no attention to the content of that choice, to how the abortion decision *ought* to be made, is not a serious moral doctrine. This is especially troubling to someone like me, who associates himself with the pro-choice movement but believes that the case for "safe and legal" abortion must be argued on moral as well as sociopolitical grounds.

It is possible to respond to this challenge by conceding its main point: that "choice" and "morality" are separate concepts, that many of the abortions now taking place in this country are immoral, but that for a variety of other reasons abortion ought to remain legal. Indeed, some pro-choice activists are now taking this tack.[1] I would be happier with a different approach. I want to make a moral argument on behalf of the pro-choice movement. I want it to be a serious argument, that is, it should not ignore the fact that many legal abortions are morally un-justifiable; it will nonetheless contend that freedom of choice in abortion is a morally defensible doctrine. As a Jew, I want to base this argument on the lessons drawn in the Jewish legal tradition, although I believe that those lessons can speak as well to others who do not share in that tradition.

I begin with the fundamental question: Is feticide tantamount to murder? The opponents of abortion rights often say that it is, and if they are correct, their argument is morally invincible. No consideration of the mother's welfare could possibly warrant the murder of her child,[2] and the state would be morally remiss if it did not extend its protection to the embryo. Yet we learn in the *halakhah*, the Jewish legal tradition, that the destruction of the fetus is not murder. The biblical text that speaks directly to the subject (*Ex.* 21:22–23) exempts from capital liability one who causes a woman to miscarry. In rabbinic law, the killing of a day-old infant is a capital offense while the killing of a fetus is not.[3] The embryo is not considered a *nefesh*, a legal person, until it has emerged from the womb; hence the essential distinction between feticide and infanticide.[4] The conclusion that abortion does not constitute murder does not mean that the fetus has no claim to our protection. As we shall see, under *halakhah* abortion may be stringently prohibited on other grounds. It does, however, tend to shift the moral burden of proof to the antiabor-tion side. Opponents of abortion cannot merely posit that abortion means the murder of babies; they must prove that the fetus *is* a "person" in order to sustain the assertion that it enjoys an absolute "right to life" and that its protection supersedes virtually all competing interests on the part of the mother. I suspect they cannot do this without resorting to theological arguments that, by their nature, are not of much help in a moral debate against adversaries of differing religious perspectives.[5]

Even if we grant that abortion is not murder, we might still have a moral obligation to protect the lives of *potential* persons. The fetus, if not a person, is surely a person in becoming; it ought not to be destroyed without compelling reason. What then constitutes a morally valid war-rant for abortion? When we turn to rabbinic law, we find that the *Mish-nah* explicitly permits abortion when childbirth endangers the mother's life. Until it has emerged from the womb, the fetus may be sacrificed on the mother's behalf.[6] Some leading halakhic authorities, apparently in-cluding the twelfth-century R. Moses Maimonides, would restrict abor-tions to such life-threatening situations.[7] This limitation is based on the talmudic discussion of abortion during childbirth, which seems to com-pare the fetus to the *rodef*, the "pursuer" who may be killed in order to save the life of his intended victim.[8] Other authorities, however, explain the permit for the therapeutic abortion on the grounds that the fetus is not a *nefesh* and that the mother's life therefore takes precedence over its own. According to their understanding, the Talmud in fact rejects the comparison of the fetus to the pursuer.[9] A number of rabbinic scholars point to an essential difficulty in the pursuer argument adopted by Maimonides. If the fetus sacrifices its right to life because it is a *rodef*, why is abortion permitted only while it is *in utero*? Does the fetus not continue to endanger the mother following emergence?[10] Moreover, how can we seriously classify the fetus as a "pursuer" when it has no intent to kill and when the danger it poses to the mother is a result of purely natural processes?[11] Some authorities simply reject Maimonides' analogy outright. They hold that the permit for abortion can be explained only through an essential distinction drawn between the mother and the fetus, by the fact that until it emerges from the womb, the fetus is not a full person enjoying a status equal to that of the mother.[12] Others through the centuries have sought to uphold the analogy, but their efforts to do so definitely cut both ways. Depending on the explanations they offer for Maimonides, these theoretical defenses can support either a very stringent or a somewhat more lenient halakhic approach to the question of abortion.[13] It is hardly surprising, then, that both approaches are amply represented in the literature. According to one view, abortion is allowed only in order to save the life of the mother,[14] and it would appear that the majority opinion among contemporary Orthodox rabbis and halakhic scholars tends toward this stringent position. On the other hand, a significant trend toward a more lenient view exists as well. A classic opinion in this camp is that of the seventeenth-century Rabbi Yosef Trani, who permits abortion for the sake of *refu'ah*, the mother's "healing," even though her life is not at risk. He rules that the fetus is not a legal person. Abortion is not murder; it is prohibited solely on the grounds that it constitutes *habalah*, physical harm to the mother, and this prohibition may be waived when her health is at stake.[15] During the present century, abortion in less than life-threatening situations has been allowed by a number of leading rabbinic authorities. The former Sefardic Chief Rabbi of Israel, Ben-Zion Meir Hai Uziel, permits abortion in order to forestall possible damage to a woman's health and the emotional stress that would follow in its wake. R. Yehiel Ya 'akov Weinberg, who headed the Hildesheimer *Rabbinerseminar* in Berlin until it was closed by the Nazi regime, rules that abortion is in order when a pregnant woman contracts rubella. R. Eliezer Yehudah Waldenberg, a renowned contemporary authority on medical *halakhah*, allows abortion when amniocentesis reveals that the embryo is afflicted with Tay-Sachs disease.[16] The issue in these latter cases, once again, is the desire to spare the mother from severe emotional suffering.

We see, then, a sharp division within halakhic thought over the grounds that justify abortion. A fascinating attempt to resolve this dispute once and for all was made in 1978, when the late R. Moshe Feinstein, a preeminent rabbinic legal scholar, published a responsum declaring that abortion is permissible only in cases of danger to the mother's life. He explicitly rejected the opposing view that, as we have seen, allows abortion in a wider range of circumstances. He thus had to account for halakhic literary sources that support the more lenient position. With respect to two crucial passages, his solution was to conclude that they simply do not exist; the one, he asserted, is a scribal error, the other a forgery.[17] Unfortunately, he supplied no proof for these assertions. This brought a stinging rebuke from Waldenberg, who condemned Feinstein's tactic in language not often encountered in this literature.[18] To erase valid evidence in such a cavalier manner merely because it is inconvenient to one's opinion is a high-handed shortcut that distorts the process of free inquiry. Such is the risk one runs when seeking to invalidate a line of thought and practice that enjoys a time-honored pedigree within a religious–legal tradition.

From the discussion in the halakhic literature, I believe, we learn three things. First, serious and principled disagreement can exist over the acceptable grounds for abortion, even among the sages and scholars of a single religious tradition. Second, efforts to resolve a principled moral disagreement, to declare one side the winner by arbitrary means, may place an intolerable strain on the very process of moral decision making. Third, the morality of any particular decision for abortion must be judged on a case-by-case basis. Danger to the mother's life is not the only moral justification for abortion. Other considerations, including her physical health and emotional well-being, are morally significant and may warrant the termination of pregnancy.[19] Whether such considerations outweigh the interests of the fetus can be determined only in confrontation with the needs of this mother in this particular situation. As a treatise on medical *halakhah* puts it, "in each and every instance, even one which seems obvious, it is necessary to consult a competent rabbinic authority [as to whether an abortion is permitted]."[20] In the here and now of this situation, her religious tradition or her conscience will demand of a woman the conclusion that an abortion is morally justified, even though well-meaning observers, judges, and legislators may disagree. The interests of morality are served and not frustrated when we allow her to make that decision. It is an odd form of morality that strips the individual of her power to choose a morally justifiable action. Yet that is precisely what happens when we operate under the misconception that morality is synonymous with the restriction of choice.

The attempt to restrict choice, although made in the name of morality, subjects what ought to be a moral decision to the control of political calculation. It is difficult to overemphasize the importance of this point. As long as the abortion debate is centered within our political institutions, there is little chance that either side will be able to move toward what Dr. Callahan terms a tougher, morally nuanced stance. Such a development requires honest, serious moral debate, and while our state legislatures are good at many things, serious moral debate is not one of them. What is going on in our legislatures has nothing to do with moral argument; the two sides have long ceased trying to convince each other through reasoned discourse. It has everything to do with the mobilization of political power. Considerations of right and wrong necessarily give way to considerations of popularity and electability. The same politicians and candidates for office, who not long ago were running for cover from the antiabortion groups, are now running for cover from the abortion-rights groups that have been galvanized into political action by the *Webster* decision. This is as it should be. Politics is the mother tongue of our governmental institutions, which speak the language of morality with a strange and foreign accent. When they address the subject of abortion, though they make liberal use of the moral vocabulary, it is politics they are speaking.

Dr. Callahan is undoubtedly correct in his prediction that, in the post-*Webster* era, compromise and accommodation are inevitable. It may prove the better part of valor for pro-choice advocates to accept reasonable restrictions on abortion in order to arrive at that "middle ground that will be acceptable to public opinion" (p. 68). Although these may be reasonable political compromises, however, they will be just that: political compromises. They will emerge out of hard-nosed negotiation, deals struck in committee, and the conscientious consultation of public opinion polls. They will partake more of concern for electoral survival than of earnest discussion of right against wrong. For example, a possible result of these compromises will be that a woman's right to abortion will differ, depending on whether she lives in Mississippi or Massachusetts. Her access to abortion will differ, depending on whether she is rich or poor, comes from an upper middle-class suburb or the inner city. Applications for abortion may be submitted to the approval of blue-ribbon panels of physicians, clergy, and other upstanding citizens who will be selected, of course, through the process of political wrangling and contention. Each of these reasonable compromises is vulnerable to charges of social injustice. Their adoption, an inescapable result of the politicization of the abortion issue, will hardly advance the cause of morality. Let us not confuse these compromises with serious moral debate. If you want serious moral debate over abortion, you should keep it away from the politicians.

Perhaps the greatest disservice that politics performs for morality is that of oversimplification. Jewish law, as we have seen, teaches that the decision for or against abortion involves a delicate balance drawn within a complex of factors between the interests of mother and fetus. Although that is a morally defensible description of how the choice ought to be made, it does not fit on a bumper sticker, and it makes a bad sound bite. As long as abortion remains a political issue, it is unlikely that the debate will ever advance beyond placards and slogans. Confronting a resolute and determined foe convinced of its moral rightness and not particularly interested in compromise and accommodation, the pro-choice movement will probably continue to respond in kind; it will have little incentive to abandon the pluralistic proposition, its own version of absolutism, in favor of a morally nuanced but politically mushy "middle ground."

It is my naive but fervent wish that the abortion question would disappear from the political arena. At that moment both sides would be free to turn their attention to the pressing moral agenda that Dr. Callahan has presented: serious efforts to reduce the number of abortions and unplanned pregnancies, to provide adequate counseling and other services for pregnant women, and to remedy the scandalous lack of social support and services for women and their children. Religious leaders in particular, relieved of the onerous burden of testifying before legislative committees and organizing demonstrations at the several state capitols, would be able to address themselves to the task of moral education, of providing individuals on both sides of the debate and in its middle with the ethical tools to distinguish between good and bad reasons for abortion. This is the agenda of moral seriousness, the only agenda that can inject a note of civility and usefulness into the cacophonous abortion debate. It will not assume center stage unless and until that debate enters a new stage, when efforts to restrict through legislation a woman's freedom to choose either cease or are defeated.

The moral argument for pro-choice, then, is not the pluralistic proposition, which Dr. Callahan rightly terms a "thin and minimalistic, relativistic idea of personal morality" (p. 58). Advocates of abortion rights need not claim that the abortion decision is morally irrelevant or that every abortion is morally justified. Their argument is rather that the abortion decision must be made by the individual in a context of freedom if it is to have any claim to moral integrity. To do otherwise is to substitute a particular view of morality for morality itself or, as Dr. Callahan puts it, to assume to have "solved a moral problem that has . . . never found any single historical solution" (p. 66). He is most assuredly right: Free choice is not the same thing as morally serious choice. The advocates of choice would do well to heed his advice to move beyond the pluralistic proposition. They would simply point out that we distort morality when we deny a woman the opportunity to reach what in her particular situation is a morally justifiable decision. Free choice is the best, indeed the only insurance that this will not happen, that the ends of morality will be served and that the decision for abortion will be, in its fullest sense, honestly and seriously made. For this reason, it seems to me, pro-choice is a morally defensible position.

NOTES AND REFERENCES

1. See Ruth Anna Putnam, "Being Ambivalent About Abortion," *Tikkun* 4 (September/October 1989): 81–82.

2. "If a person be told:" 'violate this commandment of the Torah and your life will be spared,' let him transgress and not be killed, except for the sins of idolatry, sexual immorality, and murder." The Babylonian Talmud [b.], Tractate Sanhedrin fol. 74a. [A complete English translation of all talmudic references is available in *The Babylonian Talmud*, R. Isidore Epstein, ed. (London: Soncino Press, 1969)—Ed.] See also R. Mosheh b. Maimon (Maimonides), *Mishneh Torah*, Hilkhot Yesodei Ha-Torah 5: 1–3. [A complete English translation of this part of Maimonides' code may be found in *The Mishneh Torah of Maimonides: Book I*, Moses Hyamson, ed. (New York: 1937)—Ed.] Cf. Joseph Karo, *Shulḥan Arukh*, Yoreh De'ah 157:1.

3. *Mishnah* [M.], Niddah 5:3 [A complete English translation of all passages from the *Mishnah* may be found in *The Mishnah: A New Translation*, Jacob Neusner, ed. and trans. (New Haven: Yale University Press, 1988)—Ed.] (See R. Yom Tov Lippman Heller's commentary *Tosafot Yom Tov* and R. Israel Lipschutz's *Tiferet Yisrael ad loc.*), b. Niddah 44b, and the tannaitic midrash, *Sifra*, Emor, ch. 20, n. 1.

4. M. Ohalot 7:6; Rashi, Sanhedrin 72b, *s.v. yatza rosho*; R. Mosheh b. Naḥman, *Ḥiddushei Ha-Rambam*, Niddah 44b; R. Menachem Ha-Meiri, *Beit Ha-Beḥirah*, Sanhedrin 72b.

5. I do not wish to enter here into a comparative analysis of other theological and philosophical conceptions of "personhood" against the halakhic view. I would suggest only that those who claim that a position that awards full personhood to the fetus is morally superior to the traditional Jewish stance must find a way to distinguish between feticide (permitted in certain cases) and infanticide (always prohibited), if they believe that abortions are ever justified. They have two choices. (1) They may allow an abortion in order to save the mother's life, on grounds that the fetus as "pursuer" forfeits its otherwise equal right to life. This position suffers from the problems attending to the Maimonidean view described below. (2) They may allow abortion under various circumstances because there exists an essential difference in status between mother and fetus. Those who choose the second option, whether or not they award the designation of "person" to the fetus, are in substantial agreement with the halakhic position.

6. M. Ohalot 7:6.

7. *Mishneh Torah*, Hilkhot Rotzeaḥ 1:9.

8. b. Sanhedrin 72b.

9. See the sources cited in note 4, along with R. Joshua Falk Katz's *Sefer Me'irat Einaim*, Hoshen Mishpat 425, no. 8, who argue that even Maimonides (as well as the *Shulhan Arukh*, which follows Maimonides here) agrees that the fetus is not a *rodef*.

10. R. Yehezkel Landau, *Noda Biy'hudah* (Prague, 1811), Hoshen Mishpat, vol. 2, no. 59, end; R. Akiva Eiger, *Ḥiddushim*, M. Ohalot 7:6.

11. *Arukh Ha-Shulḥan*, Hoshen Mishpat 425, no. 7; *Tiferet Yisrael*, M. Ohalot 7:6.

12. See *Sefer Me'irat Einaim* ad loc. Cf. Eiger, *Arukh Ha-Shulḥan* and *Tiferet Yisrael ad loc.*

13. Among the most stringent is the nineteenth-century R. Ḥaim Soloveitchik, *Ḥiddushei R. Ḥaim Ha-Levy 'al Ha-Rambam*, Hilkhot Rotzeaḥ 1:9. In his view, Maimonides regards the fetus in this case as an "imperfect" example of a pursuer; unlike other pursuers, it does not sacrifice its right to life. It may be aborted only because it is not yet a *nefesh*, a situation that holds only while it remains *in utero*. From this it follows that abortion is allowed only when the mother's life is endangered. On the other hand, the twentieth-century decisor, R. Ḥaim Ozer Grodzinksy explains that the *rodef* argument applies only to abortion during labor. Once the fetus has become "uprooted," it possesses an independent status short of personhood that can be superseded only by the fact of danger to the mother. Before labor has begun, he argues, Maimonides would agree that the fetus is "a limb of the mother" and may be sacrificed in certain grave situations even though it is not yet a *rodef*. See *Aḥi'ezer*, vol. 3, no. 72, sec. 3. The "lenient" authorities on abortion tend to adopt this kind of approach to Maimonides' ruling.

14. R. Moshe Feinstein, *Iggerot Mosheh* (Bene Brak, 1985), Hoshen Mishpat, vol. 2, no. 69; R. Isser Yehudah Unterman, *No'am*, vol. 6, 1–11.

15. See the responsa of the *Maharit*, no. 99. Trani mentions as well the mishnah and gemara in b. Arakhin 7a, which permit execution of a pregnant woman and abortion in order to prevent any untoward desecration of her corpse as support for the contention that the fetus is not a *nefesh*. R. Erusi, in *Techumin*, 2 (1981): 515–516, raises the interesting methodological argument that since b. Arakhin is an "indirect" source, dealing primarily with the penal law and not with abortion, it ought not to be applied to the latter issue. Trani, apparently, would have disagreed with this view.

16. R. Ben-Zion Uziel, *Mishpetei Uziel* (Tel Aviv, 1935), Hoshen Mishpat, 47; R. Yeḥiel Ya'akov Weinberg, *Seridei Esh* (Jerusalem, 1966), vol. 3, no. 127; R. Eliezer Yehudah Waldenberg, *Tzitz Eliezer* (Jerusalem, 1975), vol. 13, no. 102.

17. See note 15; the responsum appeared earlier in *Ha-Pardes*, 52 (1978): 7–15. The sources referred to are Tosafot, Niddah 44a–b, s.v. *ihu* [scribal error], and the Trani responsum (see no. 13, forgery).

18. E. Waldenberg, "Be-Inyan Hafsakat Herayon Le-Tzorekh Gadol," in *Hilkhot Rof'im U-refu'ah*, A. Steinberg, ed. (Jerusalem, 1978), 33–46; reprinted in *Tzitz Eliezer* (Jerusalem, 1985), vol. 14, no. 100.

19.   The halakhic sources tend to refer to such considerations as *tzorekh ha-em*, the mother's "need." This may be expressed as a *tzorekh gadol*, an "overriding" need. See R. Ya'akov Emden, *She'elat Yavetz* (Altona, 1739), no. 43. Or it may be expressed as a *tzorekh kalush*, a "thin, not-so-overriding" need. See Uziel, *loc. cit.*)

20.   A. S. Avraham, *Nishmat Avraham* (Jerusalem: 1987), Hoshen Mishpat, vol. 3, no. 425: 223.

5

Dilemmas in Fetal Research, Genetic Counseling, and Neonatal Care

Frank D. Seydel

INTRODUCTION

Nowhere do life and death issues seem more poignant and more closely interwoven than in the events surrounding pregnancy and birth. For sick fetuses, birth and death may be one continuous experience, and the loss of a wanted pregnancy or newborn is typically a profoundly saddening experience. Recent advances in medicine have greatly extended our opportunities to save and treat individuals in both the prenatal and the neonatal period, but these same advances often raise enormous questions about such issues as optimum treatment, wise use of resources, the quality of life of the treated individuals, and the chances of such problems recurring in a future pregnancy. Often, genetic counselors are key persons in consoling and in advising couples about many of these issues.

The scope of the dilemmas raised in this trilogy of issues is, for me, mind-boggling, and I do not hope in this single paper to systematically resolve all of them. In fact, I do not know how to resolve all of them. My interest in these issues, and any insight about them, arises out of the work that I do. Thus I hope that the reader will permit me to share my background with him or her, as a way of beginning an exploration for answers to these various dilemmas.

I am a biochemist and a United Methodist minister. I have always been interested in the interaction of religion and science, particularly genetics. In recent years science and religion have converged on genetics; some would say they have collided.

As a biochemist, I direct the Prenatal Screening Laboratory at Georgetown University Medical Center. The primary assay that I conduct is the maternal serum α-fetoprotein assay. This assay is a screening test for two categories of defects: chromosome abnormalities such as Down's Syndrome and neural tube defects. These two types of problems tie as the two most common serious birth defects. Each occurs with an incidence of approximately one in 750 pregnancies. Of neural tube defects there are two major types, each occurring in equal number, anencephaly and spina bifida.

I counsel women and couples regularly about genetic problems and birth defects. Most frequently, I counsel women about their adverse screening results. The definitive step is amniocentesis, a step that many couples take reluctantly because of its low but real risk of fetal loss. In addition to this counseling, I also counsel women and couples when the amniotic fluid α-fetoprotein test and ancillary tests demonstrate a serious abnormality, such as a neural tube defect, an abdominal wall defect, hydrocephalus, nonfunctional kidneys, or miscellaneous severe abnormalities. Many of these abnormalities are fatal; the rest severely compromise the health and life span of those babies that survive to term. Finally, I do general prenatal counseling for women age 35 and older, for women concerned about the effects of teratogens on the pregnancy, and for couples with a family history of genetic problems or birth defects.

As I have already mentioned, I am also a United Methodist minister. As such, I am concerned about helping people live value-filled lives. One dimension of this concern involves counseling. As I will discuss in more detail later, genetic counseling and pastoral counseling are quite distinct enterprises, yet they both share a concern for patients who must grapple with decisions that have profound ethical implications. Genetic counselors provide the medical information; pastoral counselors mediate the values and the spiritual and emotional support.

The enterprise of medical genetics has become vastly complicated recently. Indeed, only 20 years ago there was no formal training program for genetic counselors. Because the technology and the clinical practice are moving so fast, not unexpectedly we have a lag in cultural consensus and in religious response. C. P. Snow hinted at this a generation ago with his depiction of two cultures.[1] Consequently, the other overt dimension of my ministry is the codirection of a Program for Pastoral Care Education in Genetics at Georgetown. The objective of the program is to provide training and develop resources that will better enable clergy (rabbis, priests, and ministers) and concerned laypersons (e.g., pastoral care workers, chaplains, and educators) to work with their congregations and their denominations on these issues.

In the past two decades, religion and science have converged on genetics. There are three dimensions to this interaction: theological, ethical, and pastoral. For the sake of conceptualizing these dimensions, imagine that these three dimensions form the apices of a triangle. Each of these three apices can be framed as a question. The theological question is: How do we know what we ought to do? The ethical question is: What ought we to do? And the pastoral question is: How do we help people do well that which they ought to do? This triangular model has two advantages. First, one can start at any apex to address a religious question. Second, one can proceed in either or both directions from one's starting point. I am not a bioethicist. My training and experience have been in the areas represented by the other two apices, theology and pastoral care, and I hope to share with the reader insights gained from those perspectives.

Logically, we might start with the theological apex, with first principles. Prior to asking what we ought to do, it seems reasonable to ask how we are to know what we ought to do? What basic principles guide us and how do we know them? In a pluralistic society there is no consensus on these points, and many people skip these questions in frustration, rushing on to the ethical questions.

Most of the attention to date has been focused on the ethical situation. In a society focused on action, on doing things, this is understandable. Our questions arise in the doing: What ought I to do *now* regarding some particular activity in which I am involved? For examples we have questions such as "What ought I to do about the care of this seriously ill newborn?" or "How ought I to counsel this woman about abortion?" Indeed, our language reflects the locus of our concern. The neologism "bioethics" was coined not quite two decades ago.[2] Note that we do not use the analogous terms "biotheology" or "biopastoral care."

Yet the problem with starting with ethics is that in a society driven by technological change, we are always caught "in the crunch." It could be worse. As a society we do *not* do everything that we *could* do; hence we do not do all the evil that we could do. However, believing in the value of serendipity, we exercise little direction over research. Thus what is new in research sets the agenda for policy debate. The advantage of the "ethics-first" approach is that we do not waste time on hypothetical questions. The disadvantage is that we are always responding to questions after the fact. Some of these questions will require years for us to reach consensus, and on some of them we may never achieve consensus. I will look at three of these difficult ethical questions shortly: the use of anencephalic infants as organ donors, the use of fetal tissue for experimental therapy, and the development of DNA analysis for genetic testing.

My own experience of working with patients suggests that most families start at the third apex, that of pastoral care. I struggle along with families who need help—help in decision making and help in carrying out a difficult course of action when there is no apparent good answer. For us as helpers, the pastoral question is, "How do we best help people?" For the individual and the family, the questions are, "How do I do well that which I ought to do?" and "How do I make a choice by which my family and I can abide?"

What families decide that they ought to do is in large part determined by the support available and by their feelings of the ways in which various alternative actions will enhance or detract from their sense of self and family esteem. In turn, distillation of these experiences has a profound effect on their theology. Let me offer a typical, if over-simplified, example. The belief that a child's birth defect is somehow part of God's plan can be very comforting, particularly if that child is not one's own child. This belief implies that one has no control and perhaps has nothing to do about the situation. This reassuring conclusion reinforces the initial belief. In contrast, the idea that all events are due to God's plan often becomes disturbing if one's child is born with a serious congenital problem. This belief may lead to anger at God, then rebellion against God, and finally the conclusion that there is no God, or at least no God worth worshiping.

I stress this triangular or tripartite model of religious issues because of my belief that it will ultimately help us sort out some of the specific issues to be explored in this paper. I hope that this approach will help us find a path through the dangerous horns of the dilemmas that we will examine.

ANENCEPHALIC INFANTS AS ORGAN DONORS

As I mentioned at the beginning, the breadth of the overall topic is enormous. To deal with the topic manageably, I have chosen to limit my consideration to one issue in each area. Let me begin with neonatal care. One of the biggest recent controversies has involved the use of anencephalic infants as organ donors.

In the past 20 years there has been growing success in transplanting organs into adults with end-stage kidney disease and, more recently, end-stage heart disease. Although tissue (i.e., bone marrow) transplantation is currently practiced for children with leukemia and other tumors, organ transplantation has not generally been available for young infants. Nevertheless, the need for small organs is considerable. A. M. Capron has summarized these data.[3] In the United States, approximately 300 to 500 children die annually of end-stage kidney disease, 400 to 800 children die of liver failure, and 400 to 800 die at birth or in the neonatal period of congenital heart disease. Moreover, if small organ donation were to become proficient, it could replace current methods of treatment for various metabolic disorders. Thus, for example, children with diabetes mellitus might be given pancreatic transplants. Altogether this adds up to approximately 1,700 infants per year who could benefit from organ transplants in the United States alone.

The condition with the most attention in the press to date has been hypoplastic left heart syndrome, a deficient development of the side of the heart that pumps the blood to the body. This condition results in the heart being unable to circulate the blood adequately. This condition does not cause any problems to the fetus. However, immediately after birth, the ductus arteriosus closes, the circulatory load on the left side of the heart is thereby greatly increased, and the infant invariably dies. A major reason why condition has received so much attention is that babies with hypoplastic left heart are normal in every respect except for the heart defect.[4] If the heart defect could be corrected, these babies should survive and live normal lives with presumably normal life expectancies. Unfortunately, there is no currently effective surgical or medical treatment for this condition. In 1985, surgeons at Loma Linda University Hospital in California transplanted a heart from a young baboon into "Baby Fae," a baby with hypoplastic left heart syndrome.[5] The baboon heart was rejected by "Baby Fae." Human heart transplantation offers far greater hope for success.

Although many newborns might benefit from organ transplantation, few organs are available. Hearts and kidneys for transplantation are usually available only from infants who suffer brain death as a result of birth asphyxia, sudden infant death syndrome, head trauma or battering, near-drowning episodes, or other severe injuries.[6] However, organs from these infants are often unsatisfactory for transplantation due to anoxic injury to the heart and kidney as well as to the brain.

Loma Linda University Medical Center's pediatric cardiothoracic surgeon-in-chief, Leonard Bailey, proposed the use of anencephalic infants as organ donors.[7] Anencephalic infants are born at the rate of one per 2,000 live births in the United States. Thus, at the national birth rate of 3.70 million births per year, there are approximately 1,850 anencephalic infants born per year in the United States alone. Therefore, there would appear to be enough such infants to approximate the demand for donors, even considering that some of these infants may not be suitable as donors due to low birth weight and other complications. Moreover, anencephalic infants are uniquely suited as donors for four reasons: (1) additional congenital problems are rare,[8] (2) they face certain death

within 1 to 7 days,[9] and (3) because there is no consciousness or possibility of consciousness,[10] (4) pain is improbable.[11]

The use of anencephalic infants as donors is not new. Fred Rosner et
al. document numerous cases going back to 1966.[12] Altogether, however, these cases are relatively infrequent. But the demand has grown as
surgeons gain skills in working with tiny organs. Several recent cases
have highlighted this issue by receiving wide publicity in the lay press.
Rosner et al. summarize these two cases:

> On October 12, 1987, a woman from Orillia, Ontario, Canada, gave birth
> to an anencephalic daughter. The mother knew in advance of her baby's
> condition but decided to carry the child to term specifically hoping to use
> her organs to save the life or lives of one or more other children. After
> birth, the anencephalic infant breathed on her own for about 14 hours,
> when she was placed on a respirator and moved to University Hospital in
> London, Ontario. Approximately 30 hours later she was declared brain
> dead by three physicians not associated with the transplant team, who
> determined, after three separate ten-minute apnea tests, that she had no
> spontaneous respiration. After each apnea test, she was returned to the
> respirator to maintain organ perfusion and viability. The infant girl was
> flown to Loma Linda University Medical Center in California, where an-
> other team of physicians verified her to be brain dead. At Loma Linda, a
> woman whose unborn child was determined to have hypoplastic left-heart
> syndrome underwent a cesarean section. Within hours, the baby with the
> hypoplastic heart received the heart of the anencephalic baby . . . .
>
> Less than a month after the Canadian anencephalic heart donor case
> was widely publicized, another case was reported in the lay press in which
> the parents of an anencephalic fetus in Arcadia, California, allowed (or
> persuaded) physicians at Loma Linda University Medical Center to main-
> tain their baby on life-support systems so that its organs could be donated
> to save the lives of other potentially salvageable infants.[13]

Bailey also cites the emotional benefit arising from the desire of parents to salvage meaning from "an otherwise totally negative" pregnancy
and birth.[14] Certainly such an experience produces a profound sense of
loss and unfulfillment for parents. But the idea that such a pregnancy is
wasted depends on the meaning one attaches to life and on the expectation that life in general and birth in particular are supposed to turn out
well. I cannot but wonder to what extent parents suggest the idea of
salvage and to what extent Dr. Bailey might suggest the idea to parents.
Notably, in the same article Dr. Bailey has stated that anencephalic
babies are nonperson humans and "to disallow the use of anencephalics
as organ donors is to forfeit an opportunity for brain normal infants,
children and adults to live."

Ideally, the necessary organs could be obtained without harm to the
baby, that is, they could be obtained at the moment of death. Thus, there

would be no need to change medical and legal standards. Loma Linda University Medical Center, the leader in this area, adopted a protocol in December 1987, to provide ventilatory support to anencephalic infants at birth. The infants would then be monitored for up to 7 days or until all brain functions had ceased. Loma Linda modified the protocol in April 1988, attempting to increase the likelihood that brain death would occur within the 7-day limit (while the potential recipient would still be in reasonably good physical condition); ventilatory support would be delayed until the infant began to manifest major respiratory or circulation difficulties. However, the program was discontinued in July 1988, because few of these infants actually became brain dead under such circumstances.[15]

The failure of this ideal approach has led to several alternative proposals that would require amending the law.[16] The first, proposed in New Jersey, would revise the Uniform Anatomical Gift Act (UAGA) to allow removal of vital organs from live patients. The second, proposed in California, would expand the Uniform Definition of Death Act (UDDA) to include anencephaly as a variant of "brain death." The third would define anencephalic infants as nonhuman persons or nonpersons and therefore outside the scope of laws protecting innocent human life.

There are problems with each approach. Each appears to create its own slippery slope. The first alternative, that of revision of the UAGA, opens up the unsavory possibility of exempting from homicide statutes those who are about to die anyway, for example, persons in the final stages of a terminal illness after they have lost consciousness. Shewmon et al. state:

> As a result of the national interest in Loma Linda's protocol, for example, that institution received from "good" physicians several referrals of infants with less severe anomalies for organ donation, such as "babies" born with an abnormal amount of fluid around the brain or those born without kidneys but with a "normal brain." Moreover, the referring physicians "couldn't understand the difference between such newborns and anencephalics." Joyce Peabody, M.D., chief of neonatology there and primary drafter of the protocol, deserves much credit for her courageously candid statement: "I have become educated by the experience. . . . The slippery slope is real."[17]

The second alternative is the revision of the UDDA to define anencephalic infants as dead due to "brain absence." This alternative is the position of the Federal Republic of Germany.[18] However, it also has numerous problems. At the heart of the proposal is the assumption that there is no possibility of misdiagnosis. To someone who does not actually engage in medical diagnosis that seems simple enough in the case of something so severe as anencephaly. Michael Harrison, director of the fetal transplant program at the University of California–San Francisco, who proposed brain absence, contends that it "can be narrowly defined and cannot be expanded to include individuals with less severe anomalies or injuries."[19] A number of critics, however, disagree. Shewmon et al. discuss this issue at length; they point out that many other conditions have been misdiagnosed as anencephaly, from amniotic band syndrome to microcephalic encephalocoele.[20]

The risk of misdiagnosing could certainly be minimized by requiring a stringent protocol for diagnosis in those instances where transplantation is contemplated. Ultimately, however, many of these cases might go to court and it is unlikely that judges and juries will be capable of precise determination.[21] This is so both because of the technical complexity of medical diagnosis and because of the lack of familiarity of the average person with these various rare defects. Examination of the incidence statistics helps to dramatize this latter point. As was stated earlier, there are approximately 1,850 cases of anencephaly per year, out of a United States population of 251 million persons. That is equivalent to one case per 115,000 persons, which in turn is equal to less than half a dozen cases, of at most several days' existence, per year in a medium-sized city. The condition is simply too rare to provide the average citizen with a meaningful encounter.

It is foolish to assume that judges with no firsthand knowledge of the medical circumstances can successfully adjudicate these matters. However, these medical and legal difficulties are probably not compelling limitations to either proponents or opponents. After all, the assorted group of infants listed by Shewmon et al. is all imminently fatally affected. The exact diagnosis among these various fatal alternatives becomes important only if it is carelessly obtained (which is a procedural issue), or if the exact nature of the defect is not the real issue.

This last point takes us to the third alternative, that anencephalic infants are nonpersons, lacking any interest in the disposition of their fate. It is no coincidence that this is the position of the Loma Linda University Medical Center team, which has led this transplant research.[22] And this position appears to be reinforced by the action of most of the women who are diagnosed as carrying an anencephalic fetus; it has been my observation that most of these women abort.

Aside from the extremists in ethics who propose that no infant is yet a person, and aside from the diagnostic difficulties discussed above, the issue boils down to a fundamental issue in ethics and public policy: the value of the individual and the nonindividual. Setting aside the controversy over the difficulty of measuring consciousness in the anencephalic infant, at first glance the anencephalic infant seems to be a nonperson.

He is not conscious; he has never been conscious; and he does not have the potential of ever being conscious. Thus this infant is not like the persons exemplified by Karen Ann Quinlan, who lost consciousness. The ethicist Singer would suggest that

> if we compare a severely defective human infant with a nonhuman animal, a dog or a pig, for example, we will often find the non-human to have superior capacities, both actual and potential, for rationality, self-consciousness, communication, and anything else that can plausibly be considered morally significant. Only the fact that the defective infant is a member of a species Homo sapiens leads it to be treated differently from the dog or pig. Species membership alone, however, is not morally relevant.[23]

I would contend that just the opposite is true. Species membership is morally relevant. It is for sake of membership in the species that we treat the dying unconscious with respect, and it is for the sake of continuity with the species that we treat cadavers with respect. This minimum respect should also be the case for anencephalic infants, since it is impossible to determine precisely the minimum limit of humanness. It is for that reason that I have consistently referred to the beings under consideration as "anencephalic infants," not merely "anencephalics." Our language frames our way of examining issues, and the symbolism is important.

The consensus in the literature supports my position. Aside from the enthusiasts eager to obtain organs, there is little support for the endeavor. All of this is most frustrating to utilitarians. But we must explore other ways to increase the utility of the situation without compromising any individuals, either anencephalic infants or their grief-stricken parents. I will return to this point towards the end of the paper.

FETAL RESEARCH

The second issue I wish to explore is fetal research. Fetal tissue offers promise for a wide range of diseases. Because fetal tissue is relatively undifferentiated, fetal cells may have a number of possible advantages over fully differentiated cells, for example, greater totipotency, a higher rate of growth, and less immunological reaction.

Nolan summarizes the current possibilities for the use of fetal tissue in therapy.[24] The treatment of radiation-induced bone marrow failure with fetal liver cells already has been attempted; these cells could also prove helpful for treating other diseases of the bone marrow, such as leukemia and aplastic anemia, or certain hereditary blood and clotting disorders, such as sickle cell anemia, thalassemia, and hemophilia. Fetal neural cells are being considered for the treatment of a variety of neurological disorders, such as Huntington's disease, Parkinson's disease, Alzheimer's disease, spinal cord or other neural tissue injuries, and some forms of cortical blindness. In the more distant future fetal cells could even be used for treatment of various metabolic genetic disorders.

These various disorders, unfortunately, are all too common. In the United States alone, one and one-half million patients have Alzheimer's disease, one million have major blood disorders, one-half million each have diabetes and Parkinson's disease, and a quarter million newborn infants die annually from serious biochemical disorders.[25] The following poignant scenario by Mahowald, Silver, and Ratcheson reveals the potential value of such therapy in a way that numbers alone cannot:

> A fifty-year-old patient, debilitated from Parkinson's disease, is unable to work or live independently. He and his family have suffered from the economic and emotional effects of the disease. Physically, he experiences rigidity of his arms and legs; he has lost facial expressions; his extremities shake; he walks with a shuffling gait; he has difficulty swallowing and speaking. As the disease progresses, these symptoms are becoming more pronounced. Although some symptoms can be alleviated by medication, successively larger doses are required, to a point where the doses may actually trigger symptoms. Since no cure is presently available, the patient can only look forward to further deterioration and premature death.
>
> An experimental treatment has recently been demonstrated to be effective in relieving symptoms of parkinsonism induced in primates. The technique involves obtaining neural tissue from viable or nonviable fetal primates and transplanting this tissue into the brain of an afflicted adult animal.[26]

There is an abundance of fetal tissue. One and one-half million elective abortions, as opposed to spontaneous abortions, are performed yearly in the United States.[27] Eighty percent of these are performed in the first trimester, due to a desire not to be pregnant. The other 20% of abortions are performed in the second trimester, due to diagnosis of congenital malformations. To put these numbers in perspective, recall that there are 3.70 million live births in this country per year. Thus, elective abortions account for approximately one out of every three pregnancies that have progressed to 8 weeks or more. To look at the issue another way, compare the abortion rate with the United States' population of 251 million. That comparison yields one abortion per year per 167 persons. Yes, indeed, there is an abundance of fetal tissue.

The use of fetal tissue is currently permitted by the UAGA.[28] Indeed, a typical hospital consent form for abortion reads, "I also authorize the Hospital to preserve for diagnostic, scientific, or teaching purposes or otherwise dispose of, in accordance with customary medical practice, the fetal or other tissue or parts removed as a result of the abortion."[29] Women undergoing abortions have been regularly requested to authorize any use that a clinician or researcher would make of the resulting fetal tissue.

Mahowald, Silver, and Ratcheson have proposed three criteria for the use of fetal tissue, adapted from organ transplantation of live donors: (1) the donor or the donor's proxy has provided free and informed consent; (2) the burden to the donor (including loss of an organ or tissue, risk, and possible pain of the procedure) is proportionate to its expected benefit to another or others; and (3) other means of obtaining the expected benefit are not available.[30] The authors believe that these criteria are met. Actually, only the first criterion is generally agreed on; fetal tissue does indeed appear to offer unique value for therapy in a number of serious and ultimately fatal conditions.

Satisfaction of the other two criteria is highly controversial. Regarding the second criterion, the burden to the fetus can be presumed to be none only if the use of the tissue is dissociated from the means of its origin: termination of the fetus' existence. Truly dedicated utilitarians have no trouble with this separation. Indeed, they even approve of a woman's conceiving in order to obtain fetal tissue.[31] This fetal tissue could be used for the experimental therapy of relatives or friends, be given generously to needy strangers, or presumably even be sold to the highest bidder.

However, such blatant utilitarianism troubles many. Perhaps to make usage more acceptable, most proponents of fetal tissue utilization struggle mightily to separate the use of the tissue from its source. Typically, they compare the procedure to the information obtained by Nazi physicians. It is asserted that, just as good use of the Nazi medical information can be made without endorsing the unethical means by which the information was obtained, good use can also be made of fetal tissue without endorsing abortion.[32] The analogy does not hold, however. The Nazi political system was bitterly opposed and defeated. Current use of the information (by no means a uniformly accepted practice) does not promote the Nazi system. Use of fetal tissue from an ongoing system for first trimester abortions can be construed as support for that system.[33]

The first criterion of Mahowald, Silver, and Ratcheson—that of the donor or the donor's proxy providing free and informed consent—is also quite controversial. In the first place, the term "donor" itself is embedded in semantic confusion. The term is borrowed from the practice of using organs from cadavers, where the cadaver represents one who had been human and might be presumed to consent to an act, the giving of its organs, that was (1) in the best interests of the human community and (2) did not cause any harm to the (deceased) giver. Clearly, at death, however, the cadaver is not the decision-maker, or "donor"; the actual "donor" is the relative or guardian of the cadaver. Nolan suggests: "The use of the single term 'donor' for both the *decision-maker* (the one who makes the gift) and the *source* of the donation probably derives primarily from the desire to encourage individuals to sign written directives (such as organ donor cards) for themselves"[34] [italics in the original].

Using Nolan's terminology, in the case of an abortus, it is obvious that the fetus is not the decision-maker, or donor, since the fetus cannot be consulted. Moreover, since this particular decision necessitates the destruction of the fetus and is therefore inimical to its interests, its consent cannot be implied, as it might for an unconscious child or for a cadaver. Finally, it is arguable whether a woman who has elected to terminate her pregnancy is justified in acting as proxy for the fetus.[35] Nolan suggests that substitution of the word "contribution" for "donation" might better clarify the relationship.

The ultimate issue, however, is the status of the unwanted fetus. Modern society has not yet resolved this issue. We seem to be as troubled today over the concept of process as were the ancient Greek philosophers 2,500 years ago when they wrestled with Xeno's paradox. At one point a new human being is but a single cell; nine months later that being has fully developed organ systems and is ready for life, however tentative, on its own. The single cell does not seem to many to command full human rights or privileges; yet the about-to-be-born baby does. Since the transition is gradual with no obvious break-points, how can one resolve this issue? I do not hope to be able to resolve this long-standing ambiguity in this paper. Yet until this basic issue is resolved, we cannot resolve the issue of the use of otherwise useless—about to be discarded—fetal tissue for transplantation.

Nolan presents a compromise that I find most helpful. Knowing that, in fact, fetal research will continue under UAGA, she suggests limiting research to abortuses which are the result of ectopic pregnancies. There are approximately 75,000 such pregnancies per year in the United States. In an ectopic pregnancy the embryo implants outside of the uterus, and surgical removal of the resulting fetus is necessary to save the life of the mother. Without removal of the fetus, both the fetus and the mother will die anyway. Thus abortion is not performed with the intention of destroying the fetus, and the fetus cannot be saved anyway. Since there is currently no way to prevent ectopic pregnancies, the ensuing abortions will continue into the foreseeable future. Nolan suggests that only such a restriction on fetal tissue therapeutic research will free the research from association with elective abortion.[36] Thus, such a restriction maintains the crucial symbolism of the inherent (though not precisely determined) worth of the fetus.

GENETIC COUNSELING

The third area of the interwoven trilogy of dilemmas is genetic counseling. The role of genetic counselors is to provide information for decision making: decision making on the management of genetic illness, on options for prenatal diagnosis and pregnancy termination, and on the conditions and the procedures for conception. The conditions surrounding reproduction include such questions as whether or not to have children, or whether to have additional children if one or more children already have genetic problems. Current conceptual procedures include fertility treatment with possible fetal reduction following hyperovulation, and assisted reproductive means, e.g., artificial insemination by a husband or nonhusband donor, *in vitro* fertilization, gamete intrafallopian transfer, and surrogacy.

All of the above issues involve loss or potential loss: loss of a family member, loss of physical or mental capacity, loss of a pregnancy, or loss or restriction of reproductive opportunity. Families facing these issues thus require both assistance in decision making and support to endure difficult times. Ideally genetic counseling and pastoral counseling should complement each other in the accomplishment of these tasks. Although genetic counselors and pastoral counselors both use the word "counseling," the word means different things to these two groups. Thus, it is important to clarify the difference.

Historically, genetic counseling evolved out of the medical model rather than the social services or clerical model.[37] Thus genetic counselors strive primarily to provide information that enables individuals and families to make decisions about genetic and medical issues. They strive to provide nondirective, value-free, counseling. In contrast, religious counselors have no scruples against directive counseling, though in practice they may not be directive.

One might expect clergy to be intimately involved in the genetic decision making and in the support of their parishioners. However, that is often not the case. At times the family might not desire clergy involvement, fearing blame or the imposition of harsh standards; at other times the clergyperson may lack awareness of genetic and medical issues or be reluctant to become involved in controversial or discomfiting matters.[38] Therefore, often a genetic counselor may be the only professional to work with a patient, particularly an outpatient, on the psychosocial and religious dimensions of the above issues. Although their historical focus has not stressed training in psychosocial support and grief resolution, modern necessity has caused them to move into the void.

I have chosen to discuss the issues surrounding genetic counseling last because this discipline occupies a middle ground in this mix of issues. Genetic counselors are deeply involved with both the prenatal period and the newborn period. In the case of the anencephalic infant, for example, the genetic counselor will be involved (where medical care is adequate) in the prenatal diagnosis and subsequent pregnancy of an anencephalic fetus, as well as the delivery and care of the newborn anencephalic infant. Medical management of the pregnancy and/or infant, recurrence risk, and the sense of loss—all need to be explored. Likewise, the genetic counselor will be involved in decisions about second-trimester abortion for genetic or congenital defect, and he or she might well be involved in a situation as unusual as fetal tissue transplantation. Again, recurrence risk, medical management, the sense of loss, and the ethics of transplantation need to be explored.

Genetic disease is a serious medical concern. It is the fourth leading cause of death, following heart attacks, strokes, and cancer. Unfortunately, however, prenatal diagnosis to date is limited; we can identify prenatally only a few of the over 4,000 known genetic disorders.[39] However, we are on the verge of a vast explosion in prenatal diagnostic capability by virtue of recent advances in molecular genetic, or DNA, technology.

The technology involves working out the exact DNA sequence of each chromosome. There is now a whole series of related methodologies based on using recombinant DNA to identify the genes of the chromosome.[40] These include RNA and DNA gene probes, specific gene markers, and recombinant fragment length polymorphisms. Using such techniques the genes for cystic fibrosis and Duchenne muscular dystrophy have recently been identified.[41] To date the DNA research has been painstakingly slow. Complete elucidation of the human genome using the current technology is estimated to take three to five decades. In a determined effort to accelerate this process, the National Institutes of Health has just begun supporting a massive, coordinated research program, called "The Human Genome Project," to obtain this information over the next 10 to 15 years.[42]

The ultimate goal of the human genome's elucidation is treatment of genetic disease. Identification of the gene and determination of its exact chemical sequence permits each gene's protein contribution to the body, such as hemoglobin or an enzyme, to be synthesized and studied. Hopefully, then, the correct gene product could be administered to individuals suffering from deleterious mutations. Replacement of the defective protein with a normal protein should restore function and health.

Until the many problems of treatment are resolved, we will be left with the ability to diagnose but not treat a growing number of genetic disorders. I perceive that the growth in molecular diagnosis of disorders will exacerbate the frequency of three major ethical challenges that genetic counselors face: abortion, nonpaternity, and confidentiality. First, molecular prenatal diagnosis of serious or fatal conditions that have no hope of treatment will stimulate the demand for abortion. The intractable issue of abortion has already been discussed in the context of fetal tissue transplantation.

Second, molecular genetic diagnosis will lead to an increase in the identification of nonpaternity. Current genetic procedures, such as family histories and biochemical assays, suggest nonpaternity in about 10% of pregnancies. This information comes as unpleasant news for couples. They had only sought information about the health of "their" fetus; now they must wrestle with infidelity as well. Diagnosis of mutant genes with DNA methodology requires comparison of the fetal genome with that of each parent. In the process, paternity or nonpaternity is much more accurately revealed than with current methodology.[43] Thus DNA methodology will only exacerbate this serious problem. Counselors must be prepared for an increasing burden of family and marital issues.

Third is the issue of confidentiality. Geneticists and genetic counselors currently identify disorders through family histories, chromosome analyses, and biochemical assays. Determination of the inheritance pattern enables the counselor to identify other family members (either immediate or extended) at risk for either developing a late-onset condition or for bearing children with the condition. People usually want to share this information, but occasionally they prefer to withhold it due to strained relationships or embarrassment. The counselor then faces a conflict between serving his or her patient's interest and preventing harm to innocent people. Again, the growth in molecular diagnosis will increase the frequency of this problem.

The above three issues will increasingly place the genetic counselor in the middle of conflicting obligations: obligations to his or her patient, obligations to the patient's spouse and family, obligations to the potential patient, i.e., the fetus, obligations to relatives of the patient, and obligations to society. Traditionally, genetic counseling, like other medical activities, has focused on obligations to the patient, the person who presents himself or herself for counseling. However, the situation immediately becomes more complicated when a couple is involved, as is often the case in genetic counseling. Nonpaternity represents just one such conflict. And within a society that stresses individual autonomy, counseling has not focused on obligations to society either. There is concern that such a focus could easily be coercive;[44] the mandatory sickle-cell screening programs that many states offered in the 1970s failed because misunderstanding produced employer and insurance discrimination and psychological abuse for carriers as well as affected individuals. Nevertheless, this emphasis can produce a conflict with a counselor's natural desire to prevent genetic disease, and with the counselor's concern over the just allocation of scarce medical resources. There is no easy balance to these opposing obligations.

THE PASTORAL APPROACH TO ETHICAL RESOLUTION

Considering all of the various ethical dilemmas that have been examined in this paper, is there any way to maximize benefits to all without denying the rights of, and our obligations to, each individual or potential individual? Can we even find any *approach* to ethical consensus? I believe that the key to ethical family decision making lies in enhancing a family's coping success. In order to elucidate, let me return to my triangular model for religious issues that I presented at the beginning. The reader will recall that I suggested that families facing loss begin with the pastoral apex. They seek to do well that which they feel they ought to do, that is, they try to find decisions with which they can abide.

In any situation a family will seek to optimize its sense of meaning or esteem. In this context, meaning does not refer to a set of articulated beliefs, and esteem does not refer to pridefulness. Rather, meaning refers to a basic sense of who and what one and one's family is and what its place might be in the world. The term "coherence" is most helpful in this setting;[45] thus, family members seek to maintain wholeness as they try to repel threats. "Wholeness" in this context has significant interrelations with its cognates, "health" and "holiness," that cannot be pursued further at this time.

Families react to problems and the ethical dilemmas that they produce by drawing upon both external and internal resources.[46] External resources are provided by a family's support system; the system includes relatives, friends, members of the family's religious group, social workers, and health care professionals. Internal resources are those possessed by family members; they include financial, emotional, social, intellectual, and spiritual assets. A family employs these resources in ways that will minimize the family's loss of coherence during a time of insult and loss.

The kinds of dilemmas examined in this paper are so difficult for families precisely because they see no solutions that preserve coherence. Either path they take seems to present them with additional loss. And often the path that the family chooses does not have ethical consensus. A creative option that produces a new path through the previous "either–or" dilemma thus supports a family's sense of coherence and, in turn, can promote good ethical decision making. The providing of creative options is, I believe, a pastoral task. Let me outline how this pastoral approach might work in each of the dilemmas that we have examined.

Recall first the case of the anencephalic infant. There were two major justifications for using that infant's organs for transplantation. One was that it enables the family to obtain some meaning from an otherwise enormous loss. The pastoral approach would recognize that need but seek other ways of fulfilling it. Too often the couple feels that it is a failure because it did not produce a normal baby. It is important to redefine success so that the couple understands that they did not fail. This approach includes legitimating a sense of mystery of life, an awareness that not all in life goes right from our perspective. It involves what the Christian calls "Grace." The justification of the medical team for transplantation of organs from a live anencephalic infant is that the organs are otherwise wasted. Again, the pastoral approach would stress the value of each individual, even the anencephalic individual, in the eyes of God. On a broader social level, the pastoral approach would seek to generate increased funding for other avenues of research on those infants who might benefit from the transplantation.

In the case of fetal tissue transplantation, the justifications are similar. The use of tissue from the abortus allows the woman to feel some good use has come from an unwanted pregnancy. The pastoral approach would first seek ways to minimize the necessity of abortion. This might involve providing that woman more adequate financial resources such as better medical care or job training. On a broader social level, the pastoral approach would seek financial and emotional resources for pregnant women, ways to reduce unwanted conceptions, and ways to generate increased funding for alternative research on those infants who might benefit from the transplantation.

In the area of genetic counseling, the pastoral approach would seek to mediate between conflicting obligations for the counselor. This approach would encourage various parties to seek reconciliation with each other, for example, husband with wife, or relative with relative. On a broader social level this approach would strive for several things. First, it would seek ways to reduce infidelity and to promote appreciation of family ties. Also, it would seek to educate employers, insurance companies, and government agencies about genetic issues, such as the nature of carrier status and the benefits of voluntary screening programs. Third, it would attempt to allocate health care resources more justly.

The pastoral approach that has been outlined is not easy; it is comprehensive and never ending. It is not a replacement for ethics. But without the pastoral effort, ethical precepts alone will fail. The image of the Good Shepherd is a powerful image within the Judeo-Christian tradition. The Twenty-third Psalm, for example, proclaims that "The Lord is my shepherd." Since, as *Genesis* tells us (*Gen.* 1:26), we are all made in the image of God, by extension we are all also shepherds, that is, we are all "pastors," and I believe that we have an obligation to follow the pastoral approach. I would encourage caregivers to work with individuals and families to enhance their coherence. Doing so will not provide all the answers to the dilemmas that we have explored, but it will begin to make our difficult and challenging world a more humane place.

NOTES AND REFERENCES

1. C. P. Snow, *The Two Cultures and the Scientific Revolution* (New York: Cambridge University Press, 1959).

2. V. R. Potter, *Bioethics: Bridge to the Future* (Englewood Cliffs, NJ: Prentice Hall, 1971).

3. A. M. Capron, "Anencephalic Donors: Separate the Dead from the Dying," *Hastings Center Report*, 17, 1 (February 1987): 5–9.

4. D. L. Coulter, "Beyond Baby Doe: Does Infant Transplantation Justify Euthanasia?" *Journal of the American Association for Persons with Severe Handicaps* 13 (1988): 71–75.

5. L. L. Bailey, S. L. Nehlsen-Cannarella, W. Concepcion, and W. B. Jolley, "Baboon to Human Cardiac Transplantation in a Neonate," *Journal of the American Medical Association* 254 (1985): 3321–3329.

6. Coulter, *op. cit.*

7. L. L. Bailey, "Donor Organs from Human Anencephalics: A Salutary Resource for Infant Heart Transplantation," *Transplantation Proceedings* 20, 4, suppl. 5 (August 1988): 35–38.

8. *Ibid.*

9. *Ibid.*

10. A. L. Caplan, "Ethical Issues in the Use of Anencephalic Infants as a Source of Organs and Tissues for Transplantation," *Transplantation Proceedings* 20, 4, suppl. 5 (August 1988): 42–49.

11. *Ibid.*

12. F. Rosner, H. M. Risemberg, A. L. Bennett, E. J. Cassell, P. B. Farnsworth, A. M. Landolt, L. Loeb, P. J. Numann, F. J. Ona, P. H. Sechzer, and

P. P. Sordillo, "The Anencephalic Fetus and Newborn as Organ Donors," *New York State Journal of Medicine* 88 (1988): 360–366.

13. *Ibid.*, 360–361.

14. Bailey, *op. cit.*, "Donor Organs."

15. D. A. Shewmon, A. L. Capron, W. J. Peacock, and B. L. Schulman, "The Use of Anencephalic Infants as Organ Sources," *Journal of the American Medical Association* 261 (1989): 1773–1781.

16. *Ibid.*

17. *Ibid.*, 1775.

18. Rosner *et al.*, *op. cit.*

19. M. R. Harrison, "The Anencephalic Newborn as Organ Donor: Case Study and Commentary," *Hastings Center Report* 16, 1 (1986): 21–22.

20. Shewmon, *op. cit.*

21. T. Leggans, "Anencephalic Infants as Organ Donors: Legal and Ethical Perspectives," *Journal of Legal Medicine* 9 (1988): 449–465.

22. Bailey, *op. cit.*, "Donor Organs."

23. P. Singer, "Sanctity of Life or Quality of Life?" *Pediatrics* 72 (1983): 128–129.

24. K. Nolan, "*Genug ist Genug:* A Fetus Is Not a Kidney," *Hastings Center Report* 18, 6 (1988): 13–19.

25. *Ibid.*

26. M. B. Mahowald, J. Silver, and R. A. Ratcheson, "The Ethical Options in Transplanting Fetal Tissue," *Hastings Center Report* 17, 1 (1987): 9–10.

27. J. A. Robertson, "Rights, Symbolism, and Public Policy in Fetal Tissue Transplants," *Hastings Center Report* 18, 6 (1988): 5–12.

28. United States National Institutes of Health, *Report of the Human Fetal Transplantation Research Panel*, Vol. 1 (Bethesda, MD: 1988) 13.

29. A. Holder, *Legal Issues in Pediatrics and Adolescent Medicine*, 2nd rev. and enl. ed. (New Haven, CT: Yale University Press, 1985), 64.

30. Mahowald *et al.*, *op. cit.* 9–15.

31. Robertson, *op. cit.*

32. *Ibid.* See Mahowald *et al.*, *op. cit.*, 9–15.

33. National Institutes of Health, *op. cit.*, 3.

34. Nolan, *op. cit.*

35. National Institutes of Health, *op. cit.*, 6.

36. Nolan, *op. cit.*

37. S. Kessler, ed., *In Genetic Counseling: Psychological Dimensions* (New York: Academic Press, 1979), 1–15.

38. F. D. Seydel, "Ethical Dilemmas in Perinatal Care: Opportunities for Clergy Assistance," in *Strategies in Genetic Counseling I: Issues in Perinatal Care*, H. Travers and N. Paul, eds. (White Plains, NY: March of Dimes Birth Defects Foundation, 1987), 16–24. This volume appears in the series *Birth Defects: Original Article Series* as vol. 23(6).

39. V. McKusick, *Mendelian Inheritance in Man*, 8th ed. (Baltimore, MD: Johns Hopkins University Press, 1988).

40. L. P. Rowland, D. S. Wood, E. A. Schon, and S. DiMauro, eds. *Molecular*

Genetics in Diseases of Brain, Nerve, and Muscle (New York: Oxford University Press, 1989), 37–207.

41.   J. M. Rommens, M. C. Ianuzzi, B. Kerem, M. L. Drumm, G. Melmer, M. Dean, R. Rozmahel, J. L. Cole, D. Kennedy, and N. Hidaka, *et al.*, "Identification of the Cystic Fibrosis Gene: Chromosome Walking and Jumping," *Science*, 245 (1989): 1059–1065. See also J. R. Riordan, J. M. Rommens, B. Kerem, N. Alon, R. Rozmahel, Z. Grzelczak, J. Zilenski, S. Lok, N. Plavsik, *et al.*, "Identification of cation of the Cystic Fibrosis Gene: Cloning and Characterization of Complementary DNA," *Science* 245 (1989): 1066–1072 and B. Kerem, J. M. Rommens, J. A. Buchanan, D. Markiewicz, T. K. Cox, A. Chakravarti, M. Buchwald, and L. C. Tsui, "Identification of the Cystic Fibrosis Gene: Genetic Analysis," *Science*, 245 (1989): 1073–1087. Cf. L. N. Kunkel, J. F. Hejtmancik, C. T. Caskey, *et al.*, "Analysis of Deletion of DNA from Patients with Becker and Duchenne Muscular Dystrophy," *Nature* (London) 322 (1986): 73–77.

42.   "Genome's Tortuous Path," *New Scientist* 122 (May 1989): 23.

43.   K. F. Kelly, J. J. Rankin, and R. C. Wink, "Method and Applications of DNA Fingerprinting: A Guide for the Non-Scientist," *Criminal Law Review* (1987): 105–110.

44.   M. Lappe, "Ethical Issues in Testing for Differential Sensitivity to Occupational Hazards," *Journal of Occupational Medicine* 25, 11 (1983): 797–808.

45.   A. Antonovsky, *Health, Stress, and Coping* (San Francisco, CA: Jossey Bass, 1985).

46.   J. J. Gallagher, P. Beckman, and A. Cross, "Families of Handicapped Children: Sources of Stress and Its Amelioration," *Exceptional Children* 50, 1 (1983): 10–18.

6

Fetal Therapy, Anencephalics as Organ Donors, and Genetic Screening and Counseling

Fred Rosner

INTRODUCTION

Rapid advances in medical knowledge and biotechnology in the past decade require that the potential risks, benefits, and ethical considerations of such advances be carefully considered. Tampering with the very essence of life and encroaching on the Creator's domain must be reverently approached. To Jews, life is of infinite value; one moment of life is equal to a life of 70 years. Thus, desecrating the Sabbath is mandated to save the life of one who may live even for only a short while. All biblical and rabbinic commandments are set aside for the overriding importance of saving a life.

Man was created in the image of G-d; human beings are holy and must be treated with dignity and respect, both during life and after death. Our bodies are G-d-given, for only G-d gives and takes life. Recent developments in medicine and science threaten our attitude to these fundamental principles. Are we tampering with life itself by genetic engineering? If G-d's will is for a couple to be barren, may we undertake test-tube fertilization and reimplantation of a fetus to overcome the sterility problem? Is fetal research and/or fetal therapy sanctioned in Jewish law? Is man permitted to alter humanhood or humanity, or both, by genetic manipulations?

This essay focuses on fetal research in the form of medical or surgical therapeutic interventions on behalf of the fetus while it is still *in utero*, the morality (or immorality) of using anencephalic fetuses or newborns as organ donors, and genetic screening and counseling. The Jewish view on these biomedical issues will be emphasized.

FETAL THERAPY AND FETAL SURGERY

Fetal therapy and fetal surgery can correct a variety of disorders and malformations, such as hydronephrosis and hydrocephalus. The International Fetal Surgery Registry reported that between 1982 and 1985, 73 placements of catheter shunts for fetal obstructive uropathy and 44 drainage procedures for obstructive hydrocephalus were performed.[1] The attempts to decompress the obstructed fetal urinary tracts resulted in the survival of 30 fetuses (41%). Pulmonary hypoplasia was the major cause of death in both treated and untreated fetuses.

J. C. Fletcher points out four ethical issues in fetal therapy and fetal surgery.[2] The first is the conflict between the perceived interests of the fetus with a correctable defect and the interests of the parents, especially the mother, who must give consent for the fetal medical or surgical intervention. The second ethical issue concerns the apparent inconsistency of encouraging fetal therapy, on the one hand, by considering the fetus as a "patient" and respecting parental choice about abortion, on the other. The third ethical issue concerns the proper conditions for learning about the fetus as an object of therapy, i.e., ethical guidelines for fetal research. The final issue is the question of the social and economic priority that should be assigned to investigations of the risks and benefits of fetal therapy.

In a later paper, Fletcher asserts that informed consent for fetal therapy may be more difficult to obtain from the parents than in other health care situations.[3] The affected fetus is nearly always a wanted child. Many parents are morally opposed to abortion, especially when fetal therapy is offered as an alternative, however risky the procedure. Thus, a careful consent process should be designed and implemented.

Fletcher also discusses two long-term issues. What is society's obligation to protect the treatable, nonviable human fetus? The ethics of abortion and the ethics of fetal therapy will collide. Abortion gives the mother's interests precedence when these are in conflict with those of a nonviable fetus. The ethics of fetal therapy, however, require society to protect the treatable, viable fetus. Further, is fetal therapy worth the costs of development for wide use? Will the correction of fetal disorders simply preserve more genetic disorders in the population and add to the burden of suffering? Fletcher concludes that the benefits to society are indeed richer than the economic savings of not performing fetal therapy.

S. Elias and G. J. Annas discuss the enhanced status of the fetus in light of developments in fetal therapy and surgery:

> These innovations raise complex ethical questions about the rights of the mother and fetus as patients. If both are really patients, do both need their

own physician? Is the obstetrician to view the fetus or the mother as his patient? Usually, there is no need to make a distinction, but what if the physician believes a procedure [such as fetal surgery] is indicated and the mother refuses to consent?[4]

One of the most difficult legal and ethical issues we currently face is how to balance the rights of the mother and the medical needs of the fetus when they conflict. The basic issue is whether the fetus is a patient separate from its mother. Although many obstetricians view the mother and fetus as a single biological entity, this perception is bound to be altered in light of advances in fetal care, which clearly differentiate the fetus from its mother for treatment purposes. Moreover, most perinatologists are advocates on behalf of the fetus. Thus, advances in fetal surgery are accentuating the potential and actual conflict between maternal interests and the interests of the fetus as a patient.

Some people interpret court-ordered obstetrical interventions, such as cesarean sections, to imply that "a woman's only function is to produce healthy babies." Many women (and men) may be offended by this unwarranted conclusion. Should women be allowed to decide with impunity on a course of action (i.e., refusal of a relatively safe intervention such as a cesarean section) that may seriously injure their offspring? Does a woman not have a moral obligation not to harm her unborn child? Should a pregnant woman be allowed to drink alcohol, smoke cigarettes, or take cocaine or crack knowing full well that such behavior has serious deleterious effects on her fetus? Who speaks for the fetus? Why should the mother be the only one who decides on what is or is not done on behalf of her unborn baby?

R. H. Blanck discusses women's rights and responsibilities during gestation. He points out that the mother's right to autonomy and privacy in reproduction is fundamental, but like all other constitutional rights, it is not absolute. He quotes J. A. Robertson, who said:

> The mother has, if she conceives and chooses not to abort, a legal and moral duty to bring the child into the world as healthy as is reasonably possible. She has a duty to avoid actions or omissions that will damage the fetus and child; just as she has a duty to protect the child's welfare once it is born until she transfers this duty to another. In terms of fetal rights, a fetus has no right to be conceived—or, once conceived, to be carried to viability. But once the mother decides not to terminate the pregnancy, the viable fetus acquires rights to have the mother conduct her life in ways that will not injure it.[5]

Robertson writes that neither law nor ethics presents any barrier to the resolution of novel legal and ethical problems posed by fetal therapy such as *in utero* surgery.[6] Doctors and parents acting in good faith may use an experimental *in utero* intervention on a fetus that would be at great risk without it, but they are not legally or morally obligated to do so. When the therapy is established, a duty to use it may arise, and a mother's refusal of the intervention may be overridden by the courts.

D. E. Johnsen points out that our legal system has historically treated the fetus as part of the mother and has afforded it no independent rights.[7] In recent years, however, courts and state legislatures have increasingly granted fetuses rights traditionally enjoyed by persons. Johnsen concludes that any law granting fetal rights should not disadvantage women or in any way infringe on the autonomy of pregnant women.

The emerging rights of the unborn, where they conflict with the health and personal interests of the mother, present complex questions, especially where the rights pertaining to viability conflict with the choices of the pregnant woman.[8] The American College of Obstetricians and Gynecologists' Committee on Ethics issued a statement in 1987 asserting that "the maternal–fetal relationship remains a unique one, requiring a balance of maternal health, autonomy, and fetal needs. Every reasonable effort should be made to protect the fetus, but the pregnant woman's autonomy should be respected."[9] The statement recommends consultation with an institutional ethics committee when appropriate. "The use of the courts to resolve these conflicts is almost never warranted." A detailed review of the subject of fetal therapy and fetal surgery was recently published.[10]

The Jewish legal and moral attitude toward abortion based on biblical, talmudic, and rabbinic sources including the responsa literature has been described in detail by D. Feldman,[11] J. D. Bleich,[12] I. Jakobovits,[13] and F. Rosner.[14] In Jewish law, although an unborn fetus is not considered a full human being until it is born, abortion is allowed only where there is a serious threat to the life or health of the mother. In regard to fetal therapy or surgery, if the risk to the mother is very small, she is obligated to allow her fetus to be treated for a correctable medical or surgical condition. If the risk is substantial, the mother is not obligated to endanger her life to save that of her unborn fetus because her life takes precedence over that of the fetus.

Because an unborn live fetus is considered to be a potential human being, it must be protected from research that involves considerable risk. However, the use of the fetus or of fetal tissue, after the fetus is no longer alive, is permissible in Judaism.[15] Parents of an aborted, nonviable fetus may find some solace in donating the fetus for research or its organs for life-saving transplantation. A new related ethical issue beyond the scope of this presentation is the use not of dead fetuses but of dead adults for the performance of medical research.[16]

ANENCEPHALICS AS ORGAN DONORS

The medical literature on the use of the anencephalic fetus and newborn as organ donors has recently been reviewed.[17] Numerous arguments both in favor and against the use of anencephalic newborns as organ donors were presented at the 1987 annual meeting of the American Academy of Neurology by Ronald Cranford, chairman of the Academy's Committee on Ethics and Humanities.[18] Supporting such use are the observations that anencephalics are permanently unconscious patients, that the diagnosis can be made with 100% certainty (unlike chronic vegetative states), and that the condition is easily recognizable by parents and others. Furthermore, these patients are truly dying (unlike those in chronic vegetative states), since the overwhelming majority do not survive more than a few days. Cranford noted that some good may come to the patient's family from a tragic situation, and that certain good will result for the recipient if the transplant is successful. The health care team will also benefit from knowing that the recipient will benefit, and the family of the anencephalic may have less guilt. Finally, Cranford pointed out the social good of providing organs in view of the better techniques for transplanting organs in the very young.

On the other hand, Cranford argued that public debate on the use of anencephalics as organ donors has not yet occurred, and that the removal of organs from such newborns is the proximate cause of death and is legally homicide and ethically euthanasia. He also suggested that we let the public know that we are contemplating using organs from anencephalics even at the risk of lawsuits. He stated further that such organ use would constitute a radical departure from the whole-brain definition of death. He expressed concern that the public's confidence in medicine may be undermined since society is not yet ready for organ transplants from anencephalic newborns.

The issue of anencephalics as organ donors may soon be overshadowed by the issue of the use of fetuses and/or fetal tissue for organ donation, raising the problem of the preconscious fetus and abortion. The pool of anencephalic donors may decrease dramatically as pregnant women who learn by ultrasound or α-fetoprotein screening that their unborn fetus is anencephalic elect to terminate the pregnancy.

J. C. Fletcher, J. A. Robertson, and M. R. Harrison point out that under existing law in the United States, organs cannot be retrieved from anencephalics until brain stem function ceases, but there is no legal or ethical barrier to retrieval upon total brain death.[19] However, the criteria for determination of brain death in children and especially young infants are extremely difficult to apply,[20] all the more so in an anencephalic newborn who has no brain. In the Federal Republic of Germany, the courts accept the concept that the anencephalic fetus has never been alive despite the presence of a heartbeat[21] and allow termination of pregnancy involving an anencephalic fetus at any time during gestation. This concept had been proposed in Germany in 1980 by F. K. Beller and K. Quakernack,[22] whose article is entitled, "Termination of Pregnancy in the Second and Third Trimester for Eugenic Indication."

K. O'Rourke[23] strongly criticizes the German thesis that "anencephalic infants may be considered brain-dead" or that "the anencephalic fetus, because of the absence of brain development, has never been alive" and insists that no organs should be removed until death has been certified on the basis of clinical signs. The German investigators responded by saying that

> Because rapid deterioration of vital signs makes most anencephalic infants unsuitable as donors after death . . . we believe that there are unfortunately no alternatives at present to intubating, immediately after birth, the anencephalic infant whose parents request kidney donation, until the kidneys have been removed.[24]

These authors argue for a "morally acceptable exception" to the total brain death definition for anencephalics.

In the United States, F. A. Chervenak et al. propose that third-trimester termination of pregnancy is morally justifiable for anencephalics because the fetus is afflicted with a condition that is either incompatible with postnatal survival for more than a few weeks or characterized by the total or virtual absence of cognitive function; and, second, highly reliable diagnostic procedures are available for determining prenatally that the fetus fulfills either of the two parts of the first condition.[25]

The suggestion has been made that the law be changed to permit organ retrieval from anencephalics by legislating a third definition of death: brain absence.[26] Supporting this proposal is the fact that brain absence can be clearly defined and limited only to anencephalics, "so that individuals with less severe anomalies or injuries cannot be classed with anencephalic babies as exceptions for brain death guidelines."[27] On the other hand, babies born with hypoplastic lungs or hypoplastic hearts are also doomed to die without lung or heart transplants, but nobody has proposed lung absence or heart absence to constitute a new definition of death. Yet there is growing support for the idea that an anencephalic fetus be considered equivalent to brain dead for legal purposes to allow the family "to salvage from their tragedy the consolation that their loss can provide life to another child."[28] Amending the law to define anencephalics as dead would be a major change in legal policy and would generate enormous controversy.

Another approach is to consider an anencephalic to be a nonperson. Since anencephalic infants have no potential for cerebral development necessary for self-awareness, they are not "persons."[29] But how do we define personhood? We do not consider the absence of a face or eyes or limbs to negate a person's humanhood. Why should a hypoplastic or absent brain be viewed differently from hypoplastic hearts, lungs, livers, or kidneys? If brain transplants become feasible, would that restore the personhood of an anencephalic? We do not remove organs from people who are "nearly dead," whether they were hit by a truck, are dying of a terminal irreversible illness, or were born with a serious physical defect incompatible with life. We do not define personhood by a person's ability to speak or understand or respond cognitively to stimuli. If that were the case, permanently comatose patients or demented or psychotic or severely retarded patients would all be considered nonpersons. Yet no one has yet suggested that we "kill" all these types of patients to use their organs for transplantation.

A. M. Capron persuasively argues that proposals to use organs from anencephalic infants to meet the growing need for transplantable organs are well-meaning but misguided.[30] It would be unwise to amend the Uniform Determination of Death Act to classify anencephalics as "dead." They are in the same situation as other patients such as the permanently comatose. Likewise, continues Capron, amending the Anatomical Gift Act to permit organs to be removed from anencephalics would be unjust and would set a bad precedent. Rather, concludes Capron,

> Medical ingenuity should be directed toward finding ways to care for dying anencephalic (and other) babies so that when they become brain-dead, they can be organ donors (with their parents' permission). Medicine should not embark on a course of sacrificing living but incompetent patients for the admitted social good of transplanting organs.[31]

Obviously, aggressive therapy for an anencephalic newborn is also inappropriate. The treatment or nontreatment of severely handicapped newborns is another large topic beyond the scope of this presentation. In general, all newborns with an effectively treatable birth defect should be treated. If the condition cannot be effectively treated, such as anencephaly or severe spina bifida or a lethal metabolic defect, aggressive treatment need not be applied.[32]

Careful discussion is needed to see whether socially, medically, ethically, and legally acceptable ways can be developed for the retrieval and preservation of organs from brain dead anencephalics. Management of pregnancies involving anencephalic donors and the management of the anencephalic after delivery also need to be carefully studied. If, for example, medical maintenance is determined to cause harm or suffering in anencephalic infants, their use as organ donors might be unacceptable. On the other hand, in the absence of such harm or suffering, if viable anencephalic organs can be retrieved when total brain death occurs, their use may be ethically and legally acceptable.

In Judaism an anencephalic newborn with independent respiration cannot be used at birth as an organ donor because it is not yet dead. But there seems to be no objection in Jewish law to transplanting organs from an anencephalic baby once it no longer has spontaneous respirations and is declared dead. From the practical standpoint, it is necessary to artificially ventilate the baby when it is no longer able to do so by itself in order to maintain organ perfusion until the transplantation procedure can be carried out. If an anencephalic newborn feels no pain since pain is interpreted by higher brain centers which this baby is lacking, it seems permissible in Jewish law to attach and maintain an anencephalic infant on a respirator until it is declared brain dead by the classic criteria, e.g., absent spontaneous respirations after one or more 10-minute apnea tests. Then, the organs may be removed and transplanted into one or more recipients whose lives would thereby be saved. Without imposing any stress or pain on the patient, the prime concern of Judaism is the saving of lives. The parents of the anencephalic child may also feel a sense of accomplishment in that some good came of their tragedy.

Such permissibility to use organs of brain dead anencephalic infants for transplantation does not extend, however, to permanent vegetative state patients. Such patients may not be placed on a respirator solely for them to serve as organ donors if there is either pain or discomfort involved. One may not use one patient in this way in the servitude of another. Man is in G-d's servitude. Man cannot demand another man in his service.

GENETIC SCREENING AND COUNSELING

Prenatal screening by amniocentesis for Tay-Sachs disease in Jewish populations is strongly advocated by geneticists to prevent the birth of a baby afflicted with this lethal disease by selective termination of affected pregnancies. Such an approach may not be acceptable in Judaism since

the obligation with regard to procreation is not suspended simply because of the statistical probability that some children of the union may be deformed or abnormal. While the couple may quite properly be counseled with regard to the risks of having a Tay-Sachs child, it should be stressed that failure to bear natural children is not a Jewish legally viable alternative.[33]

The fear that a child may be born physically malformed or mentally deficient does not in itself justify recourse to abortion. The fetus has a right to be born even if it is handicapped. Only a threat to the mother's life or health constitutes sufficient reason to permit abortion in Judaism.[34] Some rabbis allow termination of pregnancy for Tay-Sachs disease because physical, mental, and emotional pain, and anguish of the par-parents are inestimable.[35]

There is considerable support, however, for screening programs for the Tay-Sachs carrier state to provide eligible clients with genetic counseling about reproductive and mating options. Even here, one should think twice before undertaking mass screening programs because of the potential psychic burden on young men and women discovered to be heterozygotes.[36] What are the psychological problems created by the information that one is a carrier for a fatal genetic disease? Should a known carrier refuse to marry a mate who has not been tested? Should two carriers break up an engagement or a marriage if they learn they are both carriers as a result of a screening program? Should a young person inquire about the Tay-Sachs status of a member of the opposite sex prior to meeting that individual on a social level? When should a person who knows he or she is a carrier tell this fact to an intended spouse? Should one sacrifice primary prevention of Tay-Sachs disease by mate selection to avoid psychosocial consequences? Is this method of disease prevention an attractive aspect of genetic screening for recessives?

One must remember that 29 of 30 Jewish people tested for the carrier state are found to be free of the Tay-Sachs gene. It is certainly desirable for these 29 of each 30 tested to have peace of mind. Is the anxiety of the thirtieth person on learning that he or she is a carrier sufficiently great to warrant not testing at all? Obviously not! However, one cannot minimize the possible psychosocial trauma to such an individual.

The social stigma of being a carrier of the Tay-Sachs gene is not fully appreciated. Misinformed and/or uninformed people may look at carriers in the same manner as patients with epilepsy and leprosy were looked at half a century ago, i.e., as individuals afflicted with a "taboo" disease, to be shunned and ostracized from normal social contact. Discrimination against carriers of Tay-Sachs disease may also occur in a variety of areas, if the experience of sickle-cell screening is repeated. Individuals found to have sickle-cell trait were dismissed from their jobs. Several life insurance companies charged higher premiums for individuals with sickle-cell trait or refused to insure them at all. Several airlines rejected flight attendants from employment in that capacity if they had sickle-cell trait. The United States Air Force, until recently, did not train black recruits with sickle-cell trait to become pilots. Job seeking was thus made more difficult for carriers of this hemoglobinopathy. Is this fate also to be suffered by people who, on screening, are found to be carriers of the Tay-Sachs gene? Total confidentiality in screening might avoid such problems and should be an essential part of all such programs.

Such total confidentiality and anonymity are provided by the Dor Yeshorim Tay-Sachs Screening Program headquartered in Brooklyn, New York. The cornerstone of the program is to prevent the birth of homozygous Tay-Sachs babies by testing boys and girls of marriageable age in total anonymity, enabling all those tested to be guaranteed that marriage with any prospective mate who was also tested would produce offspring free of this dreaded disease.

To be tested, one calls the Dor Yeshorim office for an appointment for a blood test at one of a number of cooperating laboratories. No names are asked nor recorded during the entire process. The clients are given a card with a number, which is the only form of identification used. No test results are divulged at this time.

When a marriage match is suggested, the clients or their parents ask for the test identification number of the other party just as naturally as they would ask for details about education, income, etc. They then call a special telephone number mentioning only the identification numbers of the prospective mates. If neither one, or if only one, is a carrier of the Tay-Sachs gene, the caller is told that there is no reason why the proposed match should not go forward. If, however, both prospective mates are diagnosed as carriers, the caller is advised that the match is not appropriate and that another match should be sought to avoid tragedy. The Dor Yeshorim program is provided as a public service, has tested many thousands of Jewish men and women since its inception in 1984, and has prevented several dozen marriages with potentially catastrophic outcomes.

The birth of a child with a serious congenital deformity or mental deficiency or a lethal metabolic error, such as Tay-Sachs disease, is a terrible shock to any parents. The personal decisions involved are very difficult: whether to marry, whether to have children, whether to have a further child, whether to adopt a child. For the Jewish population, not only must medical, genetic, and psychological factors be considered in any given case, but the religious attitude of Judaism toward such matters as abortion, contraception, amniocentesis, genetic screening, and procreation, to name but a few, must be taken into account.

Genetic counseling is a correct and proper exercise of man's knowledge to prevent tragedy. The existence of an undesirable familial hereditary trait must be considered when marriage is contemplated. The counselor, however, must be sensitive to the religious commitments of the patients as well as to their total health needs. Such counseling is not without hazard in that it may precipitate or aggravate anxieties concerning the meaning or interpretation of genetic information provided by the counselor.

CONCLUSION

In Jewish tradition a physician is given specific divine license to practice medicine. According to Maimonides and other codifiers of Jewish law, it is in fact an obligation on the physician to use his medical skills to heal the sick. Not only is the physician permitted and even obligated to minister to the sick, but the patient is also obligated to care for his health and life. Man does not have title over his life or body. He is charged with preserving, dignifying, and hallowing that life. He must eat and drink to sustain himself. He must seek healing when he is ill.

Another cardinal principle in Judaism is that human life is of infinite value. The preservation of human life takes precedence over all biblical commandments, with three exceptions: the prohibitions against idolatry, murder, and forbidden sexual relationships. Life's value is absolute and supreme. Thus, an old man or woman, a mentally retarded person, handicapped newborns, a dying cancer patient, and their like, all have the same right to life as healthy people in their prime of life. To preserve a human life, the Sabbath and even the Day of Atonement may be desecrated and all other rules and laws, save the above three, are suspended for the overriding consideration of saving a human life. The corollary of this principle is that one is prohibited from doing anything that might shorten a life even for a very short time, since every moment of human life is also of infinite value.

These and other principles of Judaism guide the Jewish physician in his practice of medicine. As more physicians become familiar with the Judaic principles relating to the practice of medicine, the answers to ethical queries and ethical judgments required of the physician, such as those reviewed above, become more readily available. Such answers need to be consonant with the physician's ability to practice medicine, using the most up-to-date advances in medical science and biomedical technology. However, such answers must also remain true to traditional Judaic teachings as transmitted by G-d to Moses and the children of Israel.

NOTES AND REFERENCES

1. F. A. Manning, M. R. Harrison, and C. Rodeck, "Catheter Shunts for Fetal Hydronephrosis and Hydrocephalus: Report of the International Fetal Surgery Registry," *New England Journal of Medicine* 315 (1986): 336–340.

2. J. C. Fletcher, "The Fetus as Patient: Ethical Issues," *Journal of the American Medical Association* 246 (1981): 772–773.

3. J. C. Fletcher, "Ethical Considerations in and beyond Experimental Fetal Therapy," *Seminars in Perinatology* 9 (1985): 130–135.

4. S. Elias and G. J. Annas, "Perspectives on Fetal Surgery," *American Journal of Obstetrics and Gynecology* 145 (1983): 807–812.

5. R. H. Blanck, "Emerging Notions of Women's Rights and Responsibilities during Gestation," *Journal of Legal Medicine* 7 (1986): 441–469.

6. J. A. Robertson, "The Right to Procreate and *in Utero* Fetal Therapy," *Journal of Legal Medicine* 3 (1982): 333–366.

7. D. E. Johnsen, "The Creation of Fetal Rights: Conflicts with Women's Constitutional Rights to Liberty, Privacy, and Equal Protection," *Yale Law Journal* 95 (1986): 599–625.

8. E. Raines, "Editorial," *Obstetrics and Gynecology* 63 (1984): 598–599.

9. Committee on Ethics, *Parent Choice: Maternal-Fetal Conflict* ACOG Committee Opinions, No. 55 (Washington: American College of Obstetricians and Gynecologists, 1987).

10. F. Rosner, A. J. Bennett, and E. J. Cassell, *et al.*, "Fetal Therapy and Surgery: Fetal Rights *versus* Maternal Obligations," *New York State Journal of Medicine* 89 (1989): 80–84.

11. D. M. Feldman, *Marital Relations, Birth Control and Abortion in Jewish Law* (New York: Schocken Books, 1975), 251–294.

12. J. D. Bleich, *Contemporary Halakhic Problems* (New York: KTAV and Yeshiva University Press, 1977), 325–371.

13. I. Jakobovits, "Jewish Views on Abortion," in *Jewish Bioethics* F. Rosner and J. D. Bleich, eds. (New York: Hebrew Publishing Company, 1979), 118–133.

14. F. Rosner, *Modern Medicine and Jewish Ethics* (Hoboken, NJ and New York: Ktav and Yeshiva University Press, 1986), 139–160.

15. D. M. Feldman and F. Rosner, *Compendium on Medical Ethics: Jewish Moral, Ethical and Religious Principles in Medical Practice*, 6th ed. (New York: Federation of Jewish Philanthropies of New York, 1984), 54.

16. B. S. Coller, L. E. Scudder, H. J. Berger, and J. D. Iuliucci, "Inhibition of Human Platelet Function *in Vivo* with a Monoclonal Antibody: With Observations on the Newly Dead as Experimental Subjects," *Annual of Internal Medicine* 109 (1988): 635–638. See also J. La Puma, "Discovery and Disquiet: Research on the Brain-Dead," *Annual of Internal Medicine* 109 (1988): 606–608 and A. Akabayashi, A. Morioka, and R. J. Levine, "Research on Dead Persons," *Annual of Internal Medicine* 111 (1989): 89–90 (Letters).

17. F. Rosner, H. M. Risemberg, A. J. Bennett, *et al.*, "The Anencephalic Fetus and Newborn as Organ Donors," *New York State Journal of Medicine* 88 (1988): 360–366.

18. R. Cranford, "Medical Ethics/Vegetative State," Paper Presented at the Annual Meeting of the American Academy of Neurology, April 1987, New York City.

19. J. C. Fletcher, J. A. Robertson, and M. R. Harrison, "Primates and Anencephalics as Sources for Pediatric Organ Transplants," *Fetal Therapy,* 1 (1986): 150–164.

20. Task Force for the Determination of Brain Death in Children, "Guidelines for the Determination of Brain Death in Children," *Neurology* 37 (1987): 1077–1078.

21. W. Holzgreve, F. K. Beller, B. Buchholz, *et al.*, "Kidney Transplantation from Anencephalic Donors," *New England Journal of Medicine* 316 (1987): 1069–1070.

22. F. K. Beller and K. Quakernack, "Fragen zur Bioethik: Terminierung der Schwangerschaft im II and III Trimenon aus Eugenischer Indikation," *Geburtshilfe Frauenheilkunde* 40 (1980): 142–144.

23. K. O'Rourke, "Kidney Transplantation from Anencephalic Donors," *New England Journal of Medicine* 317 (1987): 960–961.

24. W. Holzgreve and F. K. Beller, "Kidney Transplantation from Anencephalic Donors," *New England Journal of Medicine* 317 (1987):961.

25. F. A. Chervenak, M. A. Farley, L. Walters, *et al.*, "When Is Termination of Pregnancy during the Third Trimester Morally Justifiable?" *New England Journal of Medicine* 310 (1984): 501–504.

26. See Fletcher *et al., op. cit.*

27. M. R. Harrison, "Organ Procurement for Children: The Anencephalic Fetus as Donor," *Lancet* 2 (1986): 1383–1386.

28. *Ibid.*

29. J. E. Magnet and E. H. W. Kluge, *Withholding Treatment from Defective Newborn Children* (Cowansville, Quebec: Brown Legal Publications, 1985), 166.

30. A. M. Capron, "Anencephalic Donors: Separate the Dead from the Dying," *Hastings Center Report* 17, 1 (1987): 5–9.

31. *Ibid.*, p. 9.

32. R. Weir, *Selective Non-Treatment of Handicapped Newborns* (New York: Oxford University Press, 1984), 210.

33. J. D. Bleich, "Tay-Sachs Disease," *Tradition* 13 (1973): 145–148.

34. See notes 11–14.

35. F. Rosner, "Tay-Sachs Disease: To Screen or Not to Screen," in *Modern Medicine and Jewish Ethics* (Hoboken, NJ and New York: KTAV and Yeshiva University Press, 1986), 161–171.

36. M. D. Kuhr, "Doubtful Benefits of Tay-Sachs Screening," *New England Journal of Medicine* 292 (1975): 371.

7

Death With Dignity and the Sanctity of Life*

Leon R. Kass

"Call no man happy until he is dead." With these deliberately paradoxical words, the ancient Athenian sage Solon reminds the self-satisfied
Croesus of the perils of fortune and the need to see the end of a life
before pronouncing on its happiness.[1] Even the richest man on earth
has little control over his fate. The unpredictability of human life is an
old story; many a once flourishing life has ended in years of debility,
dependence, and disgrace. But today, it seems, the problems of the ends
of lives are more acute, a consequence, ironically, of successful—or partly successful—human efforts to do battle with fortune and, in particular,
to roll back medically the causes of death. Although many look forward
to further triumphs in the war against mortality, others want here and
now to exercise greater control over the end of life, by electing death to
avoid the burdens of lingering on. The failures resulting from the fight
against fate are to be resolved by taking fate still further into our own
hands.

This is no joking matter. Nor are the questions it raises academic.
They emerge, insistently and urgently, from poignant human situations,
occurring daily in hospitals and nursing homes, as patients and families
and physicians are compelled to decide matters of life and death, often
in the face only of unattractive, even horrible, alternatives. Shall I allow
the doctors to put a feeding tube into my 85-year-old mother, who is
unable to swallow as a result of a stroke? Now that it is inserted and she
is not recovering, may I have it removed? When would it be right to
remove a respirator, forgo renal dialysis, bypass life-saving surgery, or
omit giving antibiotics for pneumonia? When in the course of my own

*Portions of this article were reprinted by permission from *Commentary* (March 1990).
Copyright © 1990.

progressive dementia will it be right for my children to put me into a home or for me to ask my doctor or my wife or my daughter for a lethal injection? When, if ever, should I as a physician or husband or son accede to—or be forgiven for acceding to—such a request?

These dilemmas can be multiplied indefinitely, and their human significance is hard to capture in words. For one thing, posing them as well-defined problems to be solved abstracts from the full human picture, and ignores such matters as the relations between the generations, the meaning of old age, attitudes toward mortality, religious faith, economic resources, and the like. Also, speech does not begin to convey the anguish and heartache felt by those who concretely confront such terrible decisions, nor can it do much to aid and comfort them. Further, generalization necessarily abstracts from the special and concrete features of each human situation. No amount of philosophizing is going to substitute for discernment, compassion, courage, sobriety, tact, thoughtfulness, or prudence—all needed on the spot.

Yet the attitudes, sentiments, and judgments of human agents on the spot are influenced, often unwittingly, by speech and opinion, and by the terms in which we formulate our concerns. Some speech may illuminate, other speech may distort; some terms may be more or less appropriate to the matter at hand. About death and dying, once subjects treated with decorous or superstitious silence, there is today an abundance of talk—not to say indecorous chatter. Moreover, this talk frequently proceeds under the aegis of certain increasingly accepted terminologies, which are, in my view, both questionable in themselves and dangerous in their influence. As a result, we are producing a recipe for disaster: urgent difficulties, great human anguish, and high emotions, stirred up with inadequate thinking. We have no choice but to reflect on our speech and our terminology.

Let me illustrate the power—and the possible mischief—of one notion currently in vogue: the notion of rights. It is now fashionable, in many aspects of public life, to demand what one wants or needs as a matter of rights. How to do the right thing gets translated into a right to get or do your own thing. Thus, roughly two decades ago, faced with the unwelcome fact of excessive medical efforts to forestall death, people asserted and won a right to refuse life-prolonging treatment found to be useless or burdensome. This was, in fact, a reaffirmation of the rights to liberty and the pursuit of happiness, even in the face of imminent death. It enabled dying patients to live as they wished, free of unwelcome intrusions, and to let death come when it would. Today, the demand has been raised: we find people asserting not just a right to refuse burdensome treatment but a positive "right to die," grounded not in objective conditions regarding prognosis or the uselessness of treatment, but in the supremacy of choice itself. In the name of choice, people claim the right to choose to cease to be choosing beings. From such a right to refuse not only treatment but life itself—from a right to become dead—it is then a small step to the right to be *made* dead: from my right to die will follow your duty to assist me in dying, i.e., to become the agent of my death, if I am not able, or do not wish, to kill myself. And, because of our egalitarian tendencies, it will continue to be an easy step to extend all these rights even to those who are incapable of claiming or exercising them for themselves, with proxies empowered to exercise a right to demand death for the comatose or demented.[2] No one bothers very much about where these putative rights come from or what makes them right, and simple reflection will show that many of them are incoherent; some people, for example, claim them as part of a so-called right to privacy or autonomy, yet shamelessly insist that my claim to privacy (or autonomy) ought to *oblige* a doctor to *intervene* in my private life for the sake of ending it. Worse, since *all* of our so-called natural or human rights presuppose our self-interested and self-loving *attachment* to our own *lives*—the foundational right, after all, is the right of self-*preservation*—attempts to derive therefrom any "right to die" or a right to be made dead are not only groundless but self-contradictory.

Comparable mischief can, of course, be done beginning with the notion of duty. From the acknowledged human duty not to shed innocent blood follows the public duty to protect life against those who would threaten it. This gets extended to a duty to preserve life in the face of disease or other nonhuman dangers to life. This gets extended to a duty to prolong life whenever possible, regardless of the condition of that life or the wishes of its bearer. This gets extended to an unconditional duty never to let death happen, if it is in one's power to do so. This position, sometimes alleged—I think mistakenly—to be entailed by belief in the "sanctity of life," could even make obligatory a search for the conquest of death altogether, through research on aging. Do we have such duties? On what do they rest? And can such a duty to prevent death—or a right to life—be squared with a right to be made dead? Is not this intransigent language of rights and duties unsuitable for finding the best course of action, in these terribly ambiguous and weighty matters? We must try to become more thoughtful about the terms we use and the questions we pose.

Now I am painfully aware that talking about talk looks like a cowardly and unfeeling thing to do in the light of the tremendous burdens people face. I have no illusions about the ability of such reflections to resolve our horrible dilemmas. In fact, I have no intention here even to try to resolve them. On the contrary, I want rather to increase the difficulty by showing the dangers in sloppy and simplistic thinking, which promises, falsely, to set matters right. Before we run off to embrace a new solution, for example, active euthanasia, we should try to get clear in our thoughts about what we are doing and why.

Toward this end, I wish to explore here the relation between two other powerful notions, both prominent in the discussions regarding the end of life: death with dignity and the sanctity of life. Both convey elevated, indeed lofty, ideas: What, after all, could be higher than human dignity, unless it were something sacred? As a result, each phrase often functions as a slogan or a rallying cry, though seldom with any regard for its meaning or ground. In the current debates about euthanasia, we are often told that these notions pull in opposite directions.[3] Upholding death with dignity might mean taking actions that would seem to deny the sanctity of life. Conversely, unswervingly upholding the sanctity of life might mean denying to some a dignified death. This implied opposition is, for many of us,[4] very disquieting. The dilemmas themselves are bad enough. Much worse is it to contemplate that human dignity and sanctity might be opposed, and that we may be forced to choose between them.

Mention of choice permits me to note, in passing, that dignity and sanctity are not the only principles that have been placed before us. Indeed, the overall theme of this volume invites us to ponder "the ethics of choice." For many (perhaps most) people working in ethics today, human choice is itself a principle, a perhaps supreme principle—not just choice as a burden or a sad necessity, not just the need to make our choices *ethical,* but an ethical affirmation of human choice *itself,* i.e., autonomy, as *the* choice-worthy ethical principle. Autonomy is a seductive because flattering principle, but hardly an adequate one, especially in the present case. For how can autonomy be asserted about birth and death, those two notches that necessity carves at the ends of every human life, defying and denying the pretensions of human will and choice to self-sufficiency (as the book of *Ecclesiastes,* with its "a time to be born and a time to die," makes plain)? True, today's conventional wisdom is partly right when it claims that birth and death are now genuinely (but, I would add, only partly) under human control, hence subject to human choice—not only about when but how. Yet for myself, this burden is a misfortune, not, as it seems for some, a cause for celebration. We *may* have to accept as our lot the sad necessity of *having* to choose, say, between sanctity and dignity, but those who celebrate the principle of autonomy would have us think that we are thereby extending human self-command still deeper over dumb and indifferent necessity—even when the alternatives before choice are themselves intrinsically bitter. To explore this important matter further would carry me far afield, but as we are trying to become self-conscious about the latent meanings of our terms, I think it worth noting that it makes a big difference if we weigh death with dignity and the sanctity of life—our two substantive principles—on the scale of freedom, rather than, say, of reverence or righteousness or duty.

The confrontation between upholders of death with dignity and upholders of the sanctity of life is, in fact, nothing new. Two decades ago the contest was over termination of treatment and letting die. Today and tomorrow the issue is and will be assisted suicide, mercy-killing, so-called active euthanasia. On the extremes of both battles stand the same opponents, many of whom—I think mistakenly—think the issues are the same. Many who now oppose mercy-killing or voluntary euthanasia then opposed termination of treatment, thinking it equivalent to killing. Those who today back mercy-killing in fact agree: If it is permissible to choose death by letting die, they argue, why not also by active steps to hasten, humanely, the desired death? Failing to distinguish between letting die and making dead (by failing to distinguish between intentions and deeds, causes and results, goals and outcomes), both sides polarize the debate, opposing not only one another but also those in the uncomfortable middle. For them, it is *either* sanctity of life *or* death with dignity: one must choose.

I do not accept this polarization. Indeed, in the rest of this essay I mean to suggest the following. First, human dignity and the sanctity of life are not only compatible, but, if rightly understood, go hand in hand. Second, death with dignity, rightly understood, has largely to do with exercising the humanity that life makes possible, often to the very end, and very little to do with medical procedures or the causes of death. Third, the sanctity and dignity of life are entirely compatible with letting die but not with deliberately killing. Finally, the practice of euthanasia will not promote human dignity, and our rush to embrace it will only accelerate the various tendencies in our society that undermine not only dignified conduct but even decent human relations.

THE SANCTITY OF LIFE (AND HUMAN DIGNITY)

What exactly is meant by the sanctity of life? This turns out to be difficult to say. In the opinion of one recent commentator, it is "the view that each moment of biological life of every member of our species is of infinite value."[5] But this can at best be a latter day and derivative formulation, for it is filled with notions of only recent vintage ("biological life" instead of "life"; "members of our species" instead of "human being"; "each moment" for "life as a whole"; "infinite value"). More fundamentally, and in the strictest sense, sanctity of life would mean that life is something in itself holy or sacred, transcendent, set apart—like God Himself. Or, again, focusing on our responses to the sacred, it would mean that life is something before which we stand (or should stand) with reverence, awe, and grave respect—because it is beyond us and unfathomable. In more modest but also more practical terms, to regard life as sacred means that it should not be violated, opposed, or destroyed, and, positively, that it should be protected, defended, and preserved. (It would be a further question whether these obligations are understood as absolute and unconditional.) Despite their differences, these various formulations agree in this: that "sacredness," whatever it is, inheres in life itself, and that life, *by its very being*, calls forth an appropriate human response, whether of veneration or restraint. To say that sacredness is something that can be conferred or ascribed—or re-moved—by solely human agreement or decision is to miss the point entirely.

Yet there is further difficulty. *Which* or *what* life is sacred: only human life or animal (and plant) life also? If the latter, is animal life sacred equally with human life, or can there be degrees of "sanctity"? And, within human life, is it the individuated being, the conscious or rational being, or the whole organism simply as human whose life is sacred? Is the lineage holy, or the race or the nation or the species? Or is it not life as such but life *lived in a certain way*, e.g., the life according to the Torah, that has sanctity?

A deeper question: What is the ground or basis of life's sanctity? Does it depend decisively on a divine act, either that life was *made* by God or that He later sanctified it (as He did the Sabbath)? Or, quite apart from its origins, is there perhaps something god-like about life or human life, e.g., spirit, that calls forth awe and respect, and before which we stand somewhat as we do before the divine? More experientially, leaving all revelation to one side, is there not something "protoreligious" in the joyous experience of birth, in the horror of extinction, and in many of the astonishing appearances and doings of all living things, before which the proper response is wondering awe? What is it that makes what kind of life sacred? Just raising these questions shows how difficult it would be, philosophically, to understand the sanctity of life.

I have made a modest and so far unsuccessful effort to trace the origin of the sanctity of life doctrine in our own traditions. To the best of my knowledge, the phrase "sanctity of life" does not occur either in the Hebrew Bible or in the New Testament. Life as such is not said to be holy (*qadosh*), as is, for example, the Sabbath. The Jewish people are said to be a holy people, and they are enjoined to be holy as God is holy. True, traditional Judaism places great emphasis on preserving human life—

even the holy Sabbath may be violated to save a life, implying to some that a human life is more to be revered than the Sabbath—yet the duty to preserve one's life is not unconditional: To cite only one example, a Jew should accept martyrdom rather than commit idolatry, adultery, or murder.[6]

As murder is the most direct assault on human life and the most explicit denial of its sanctity, perhaps we gain some access to the meaning of the sanctity of life by thinking about why murder is proscribed— that is, by following up the more modest and practical meaning, namely, that life's sanctity demands our restraint. If we could uncover the ground of restraint against murder, perhaps we could learn something of the nature of the sanctity of life, and, perhaps, too, of its relation to human dignity. As a result, we might be in a better position to consider the propriety of letting die, of euthanasia, and of other activities advocated by the adherents of death with dignity.

Why is killing another human being wrong? Can the prospective victim's request to be killed nullify the wrongness of such killing, or, what is more, make such killing right? Alternatively, are there specifiable states or conditions of a human being's life that would justify—or excuse—someone else's directly and intentionally making him dead, even *without* request? The first question asks about murder; the second and third ask whether assisting suicide and mercy-killing (so-called active euthanasia) can and should be morally distinguished from murder. The answers regarding assisting suicide and euthanasia will depend on the answer regarding murder, that is, on the reasons it is wrong.

Not all taking of human life is murder. Self-defense, war, and capital punishment have been moral grounds used to justify homicide, and it is a rare moralist who would argue that it is never right to kill another human being. Without arguing about these exceptions, we confine our attention to murder, which is, by definition, unjust or wrongful killing. Everyone knows it to be wrong, immediately and without argument. Rarely do we ask ourselves why.[7]

Why is murder wrong? The laws against murder are, of course, socially useful. Though murders still occur, despite the proscriptive law and the threat of punishment, civil society is possible only because people generally accept and abide by the reasonableness of this rule. In exchange for society's protection of one's own life against those who might otherwise take it away, each member of society sacrifices, in principle, his (natural) right to the lives of all others. Civil society requires peace, and civil peace depends absolutely on the widespread adherence to the maxim "Thou shalt not murder." This usefulness of the taboo against murder is sometimes offered as the basis of its goodness: Killing is bad because it makes life unsafe and society impossible.

But this alone cannot account for the taboo against murder. In fact, the goodness of civil society is itself predicated on the goodness of human life which society is instituted to defend and foster; were this not true, the impossibility of civil peace and decent society would hardly count as such a decisive argument. A society that, quite peacefully and deliberately, commits mass suicide (Jonestown) elicits our horror and incurs our condemnation. One is led to see that civil society exists to defend the goods implicit in the taboo against murder, at least as much as the taboo against murder exists to preserve civil society.

Murder indirectly threatens to destroy civil society, but it directly destroys individuals. However valuable any life may be to the society, each life is primarily and preeminently valued by the person whose life it is. Individuals strive to stay alive, both consciously and unconsciously. The living body, quite on its own, bends every effort to maintain its living existence. The built-in impulses toward self-preservation and individual well-being that penetrate our consciousness, say, as hunger or fear of death, are manifestations of a deep-seated and powerful will to live. These thoughts might suggest that murder is wrong because it opposes this will to live, because it deprives another of life against his will, because it kills someone who does not *want* to die (and who has not committed some offense that might justify ignoring his will to live). This sort of reason would explain why suicide—self-willed self-killing— might be right, while murder—killing an innocent person against his will—would always be wrong.

Let us consider this view more closely. Certainly, there are some invasions or "violations" of another's body that are made innocent by consent. Blows struck in a boxing match or on the football field do not constitute assault; conversely, an unwelcome kiss from a stranger, because it is an unconsented touching, constitutes a battery, actionable at law. In these cases, the willingness or unwillingness of the "victim" alone determines the rightness or wrongness of the bodily blows. Similar arguments are today used to explain the wrongness of rape: it is "against our will," a violation not (as we once thought) of womanliness or chastity or nature but of freedom, autonomy, personal self-determination. If consent excuses—or even justifies—these "attacks" on the body of another, might not consent excuse—or justify—the ultimate, i.e., lethal, attack, turning murder into mere (unwrongful) homicide? A person can be murdered only if he personally does not want to be dead.

There is something obviously troublesome about this way of thinking about crimes against persons. Indeed, the most abominable practices, proscribed in virtually all societies, are *not* excused by consent. Incest, even between consenting adults, is still incest; cannibalism would not become merely *delicatessen* if the victim freely gave permission;

ownership of human beings, voluntarily accepted, would still be slavery. The violation of the other is independent of the state of the will (in fact, both of victim and perpetrator).

The question can be put this way: Is the life of another human being to be respected only because that person (or society) *deems* or *wills* it respectable, or is it to be respected because it *is in itself* respectable? If the former, then human worth depends solely on agreement or human will; since will confers dignity, will can take it away, and a permission to violate nullifies the violation. If the latter, then one can never be freed from the obligation to respect human life by a request to do so, say, from someone who no longer values his own life.

This latter view squares best with our intuitions. We are not entitled to dismember the corpse of a suicide nor may we kill innocently those consumed by self-hatred. The taboo against murder would seem to belong with the taboos against incest and cannibalism rather than with the torts of unconsented touching. According to our law, killing the willing, the unwilling, and the nonwilling (e.g., infants, the comatose) are all equally murder. Beneath the human will, indeed, the *ground* of human will, is something that commands respect and restraint, willy-nilly. We are to abstain from killing because of something respectable about human beings as such. But what is it?

In Western societies, moral notions trace back to biblical religion. The bedrock of Jewish and Christian morality is the Ten Commandments. "Thou shalt not murder"—the sixth commandment—heads up the so-called second table, which enunciates (negatively) duties toward one's fellow man. From this fact, some people have argued that murder is wrong solely because God said so. After all, that He had to legislate against it might imply that human beings on their own did not know that it was bad or wrong. And even were they to intuit *that* murder is wrong, they might never be able to answer, if challenged, *why* it is wrong; this human inability to supply the reason would threaten the power of the taboo. Thus, so the argument goes, God's will supplies the missing reason for the human rule.

This argument is not satisfactory. True, divine authority elevates the standing and force of the commandments. But it does not follow that they "make sense" only because God willed them. Pagans yesterday believed and atheists today still believe that murder is wrong. And while the latter might be suspected of being still under the influence of a morality whose source they reject, other cultures and other nonreligious thinkers line up squarely against murder. Aristotle, who did not know the revelation of the God of Abraham, Isaac, and Jacob, spoke for rationality itself when he said that the very name, murder—like adultery and theft—implies badness. In fact, the entire second table of the Decalogue is said to propound not so much divine law but natural law, law suitable for man as man, not only for Jew or Christian.

The Bible itself provides evidence in support of this interpretation, at least about murder. In reporting the first murder, committed by Cain on his brother Abel before there was any given or known law against it, Abel's blood is said to cry out from the earth in protest against his brother's deed. (The crime, it seems, was a crime against blood and life, not against will, human or divine.) And Cain's denial of knowledge ("Am I my brother's keeper?") seems a clear indication of guilt: If there were nothing wrong with murder, why hide one's responsibility? A "protoreligious" dread accompanies the encounter with death, especially violent death. But the best evidence comes shortly afterward, in the story of the covenant with Noah: The first law against murder is explicitly promulgated for all mankind united, well before there are Jews or Christians or Muslims. This passage is worth looking at in some detail because, unlike the enunciation of the sixth commandment, it offers a specific reason why murder is wrong.[8]

The prohibition of murder—or, to be more precise, the institution of retribution for shedding human blood—is part of the new order following the Flood. Before the Flood, human beings lived in the absence of law or civil society. As the population grew, and human contacts increased, violence erupted as men helped themselves to whatever they could with impunity seize from each other. The result appears to be something like what Hobbes called the state of nature—itself defined as the state of anarchy, a state of lawlessness without any ruling power to keep the peace—characterized as a condition of war of each against all. Might alone makes right, and no one is safe. The Flood washes out human life in its natural state; immediately after the Flood, some form of law and justice is instituted, and nascent civil society is founded. Thus, the Flood represents that watershed in human affairs that separates anarchy and the coming of law and right.

At the forefront of the new order is a newly articulated respect for human life,[9] expressed in the announcement of the punishment for homicide:

> Whoso sheddeth man's blood, by man shall his blood be shed; for in the image of God made He man. (*Genesis* 9:6)

Like law in general, this cardinal law combines speech and force. The threat of capital punishment stands as a deterrent to murder and hence provides a motive (negative) for obedience. But the measure of the punishment is instructive. By equating a life for a life—*no more* than a life for a life, and the life only of the murderer, not also of his wife and children—the threatened punishment implicitly teaches the *equal* worth of each human life. Such equality can be grounded only in the equal *humanity* of each human being. Against our own native self-preference, and against our tendency to overvalue what is our own, blood-for-blood conveys the message of universality and equality.

But murder is to be avoided not only to avoid the punishment. That may be a motive, which speaks to our fears; but there is also a reason, which speaks to our minds and our loftier sentiments. The fundamental reason that makes murder wrong—and that even justifies punishing it homicidally!—is man's divine-like status.[10] Not the other fellows' unwillingness to be killed, not even (or only) our desire to avoid sharing his fate, but *his*—any man's—*very being* requires that we respect his life. Human life is to be respected more than animal life because man is more than an animal; man is said to be god-like.[11] Please note that the *truth* of the Bible's assertion does *not* rest on biblical authority: Man's more-than-animal status is in fact performatively proved whenever human beings quit the state of nature and set up life under such a law, which exacts just punishment for shedding human (i.e., more-than-animal) blood. The law that establishes that men are to be law-abiding both insists on, and thereby demonstrates the truth of, the superiority of man.

The more-than-animal status of human beings has been claimed or asserted by many traditions. Attributing even god-like standing is not peculiarly biblical; several of the Greeks, for example, suggested that man was that impossible chimera of god-in-beast. To learn what *Genesis* means by "image of God," we must probe further in this text.

The Hebrew word translated "image" is *tselem*, from a root meaning "to cut off," "to chisel"; *tselem*, something cut or chiseled out, in the first instance a statue, becomes, derivatively, any image or likeness or resemblance, something which both *is* and *is not* what it resembles. Although being merely a likeness, an image not only resembles but also points to, and is dependent for its very being on, that of which it is a image.

How is man god-like? One possibility, of course, is that man and God are alike in looks; the Olympian gods of ancient Greece were anthropomorphic, and differed from human beings only in being ageless and immortal. But *Genesis* 1—where it is first said that man is created in God's image—offers no hint of God's corporeality. Instead, in the course of recounting His creation, the text introduces us to the divine *activities* and *powers:* (1) God speaks, commands, names, and blesses; (2) God makes and makes freely; (3) God looks at and beholds the world; (4) God is concerned with the goodness or perfection of things; (5) God addressed solicitously other living creatures. In short, God exercises speech and reason, freedom in doing and making, and the powers of contemplation, judgment, and care.

Doubters may wonder whether this is truly the case about God—after all, it is only on biblical authority that we regard God as possessing these powers and activities. But it is certain that we human beings have them, and that they lift us above the plane of a merely animal existence. Never mind for now where these powers came from; their presence, and the difference they make for human life, is indisputable. Human beings, along among the earthly creatures, speak, plan, create, contemplate, and judge. Human beings, alone among the creatures, can articulate a future goal and bring it into being by their own purposive conduct. Human beings, alone among the creatures, can think about the whole, marvel at its articulated order, and feel awe in beholding its grandeur and in pondering the mystery of its source.

A complementary, preeminently moral, gloss on "image of God" is provided—quite explicitly—in *Genesis* 3, at the end of the so-called second creation story:

> Now the man is become *like one of us* knowing good and bad (3:22). [emphasis added].[12]

Human beings, unlike the other animals, distinguish good and bad, have opinions and care about their difference, and constitute their whole life in the light of this distinction. Animals may suffer good and bad, but they have no notion of either. Indeed, the very pronouncement "Murder is bad" constitutes proof of *this* god-like quality of human beings.

In sum, man has special standing because he shares in reason, freedom, judgment, and moral concern, and, as a result, lives a life freighted with moral self-consciousness. Speech and freedom are used, among other things, to promulgate moral rules and to pass moral judgments, first among which is that murder is to be punished in kind because it violates the dignity of such a moral being. We note a crucial implication. To put it simply, the *sanctity* of human life rests absolutely on the *dignity*—the god-like-ness—of human beings.

Yet man is, at most, only god*ly;* he is not God or a god. To be an image is also to be *different* from that of which one is an image. Man is, at most, a *mere* likeness of God. With us, the seemingly godly powers and concerns described above occur conjoined with our animality. We are also flesh and blood—no less than the other animals. God's image is tied to blood, which is the life.

The point is crucial, and stands apart from the text that teaches it: Everything high about human life—thinking, judging, loving, willing, acting—depends absolutely on everything low—metabolism, digestion, circulation, respiration, excretion. In the case of human beings, "divinity" needs blood—or "mere" life—to sustain itself. And because of what it holds up, human blood—that is, human life—deserves special respect, beyond what is owed to life as such: The low ceases to be the low. (Modern physiological evidence could be adduced in support of this thesis: In human beings, posture, gestalt, respiration, sexuality, and fetal and infant development, among other things—all show the marks of the co-presence of rationality.) The biblical text elegantly mirrors this truth about its subject, subtly merging both high and low: Though the *reason* given for punishing murder concerns man's *godliness*, the *injunction* itself concerns man's *blood*. Respect the god-like; don't shed its blood! Respect for anything *human* requires respecting *everything* human, requires respecting *human being* as such.

We have found, I believe, what we were searching for, a reason immanent in the nature of things for finding fault with taking human life, apart from the needs of society or the will of the victim. True, the account I have offered is abstract and cold, and hardly commensurate with the horror we feel at the sight (or news) of a murder (or even at the sight of a corpse). Yet that horror, utterly reasonable and fitting, bespeaks the same point: The wanton spilling of human blood is a violation and a desecration, not only of our laws and wills but *of being itself*.

We have also found the ground for repudiating the opposition between the sanctity of life and human dignity. Each rests on the other. Or, rather, they are mutually implicated, as inseparable as the concave and the convex. Those who seek to pull them apart are, I submit, also engaged in wanton, albeit intellectual, violence.

Unfortunately, the matter cannot simply rest here. Though the principle seems well established, there is a difficulty, raised, in fact, by the text itself. How can one assert the inviolability of human life and, in the same breath, insist that human beings deliberately *take* human life to punish those who shed human blood?[13] There are, it seems, sometimes good reasons for shedding human blood, notwithstanding that man is in God's image. We have admitted the dangerous principle: Humanity, to uphold the dignity of the human, must sometimes shed human blood.

Bringing this new principle to the case of euthanasia, we face the following challenge to the prior, and more fundamental, principle "shed no human blood": What are we to think when the continuing circulation of human blood no longer holds up anything very high, when it holds up little more—or even *no* more—than metabolism, digestion, circulation, respiration, and excretion? What if human godliness appears to be humiliated by the degradation of Alzheimer's disease or paraplegia or rampant malignancy? And what if it is the well-considered aspiration of the "god-like" to put an end to the humiliation of that very godliness, to halt the mockery that various severe debilities make of a *human* life? Are there here to be found other exceptions to our rule against murder, in which the dignity of a human life can (only?) be respected by ending it?

The first thing to observe, of course, is that the cases of euthanasia (or suicide) and capital punishment are vastly different. One cannot by an act of euthanasia deter or correct or obtain justice from the "violator" of human dignity; senility and terminal illness are of natural origin and can be blamed on no human agent. To be precise, these evils may in their result undermine human dignity, but, lacking malevolent intention, cannot be said to insult it or deny it. They are reasons for sadness, not in*dign*ation, unless one believes, as the tyrant does, that the cosmos owes him good and not evil and exists to satisfy his every wish. Moreover, one does not come to the defense of diminished human dignity by finishing the job, by annihilating the victims. Human dignity would be no more vindicated by euthanizing patients with Alzheimer's disease than it would be by executing as polluted the victims of rape.

Nevertheless, the question persists, and an affirmative answer remains the point of departure for the active euthanasia movement. Many who fly the banner of "death with dignity" insist that it centrally includes the option of active euthanasia, especially when requested. To respond more adequately to this challenge, we need first a more careful inquiry into "death with dignity."

DEATH WITH DIGNITY

As we did with "sanctity of life," we begin by recognizing the different ways people use the notion "death with dignity." We are especially well advised to notice both for whom and for what it is being asserted. Most often it is claimed on behalf of the already and actually dying, people with fatal illnesses, usually in their terminal stages. Thus, "death with dignity" is meant to address the need to protect already *dying patients* from useless or burdensome interventions that prolong their dying or that threaten to destroy the goodness of their remaining life, i.e., the problem of medical excess. But, sometimes, "death with dignity" is claimed on behalf of people who are *not* dying, but who suffer chronic, severely disabling, and degrading illnesses (e.g., Alzheimer's disease). Here, death with dignity is meant to address the wish (usually of persons other than the victim) to end the misery and humiliation of reduced humanity; since these people, unlike the first group, are *not* already dying, they need to be made dead by active killing, which, generally, they cannot do for themselves and are not even able to request. One cannot exaggerate the importance of keeping distinct the status and condition of these two groups.

But the slogan "death with dignity" is sometimes used to make claims less about dying and more about living. It means to address the need to provide a *better* way of *living* (while declining and/or dying) for those both with and without fatal illness or incapacitating disability, indeed, for everyone who ventures into old age. Dying with dignity really pleads for a dignified old age, which in turn seems to be no different from *living* with dignity, at any time of life. "Life with dignity" is, of course, in need of explication; for example, for some people, living with dignity means living *well*, for others living *as one chooses*. The latter might be said to encompass choosing the manner and timing of one's death, and it is to serve this partial purpose that a right to a death with dignity is sometimes asserted, specifically to keep the state and the criminal law from blocking access to a death of one's own devising. Finally, death with dignity is sometimes a plea for respectful *personal* treatment from others, despite one's disabilities, and is meant to address the need to preserve a precarious respect for human life as such, in the face of judgments, made by others, that the life in question is not worth living. In our political discourse, the slogan "death with dignity" addresses a multitude of purposes—allowing to die, avoiding indignities, living well in old age, autonomy, respect for the disabled—and for a variety of putative beneficiaries—who, it is worth noting, are usually *not* the people advancing the claim, which generally is made by self-appointed proxies speaking on their behalf. These ambiguities should make us wary and attentive. They also invite us to attempt a further analysis on our own.

The phrase "death with dignity," whatever it means precisely, certainly implies that there are more and less dignified ways to die. The demand for death with dignity arises only because more and more people are encountering in others and fearing for themselves or their loved ones the death of the less dignified sort. This point is indisputable. The *possibility* of dying with dignity can be diminished or undermined by many things, for example, by coma or senility or madness, by unbearable pain or extensive paralysis, by ignorance or cowardice, by isolation or rejection, by institutionalization or destitution, by sudden death, as well as by excessive or impersonal medical interventions directed toward the postponement of death. It is the impediments connected with modern medicine that increasingly arouse indignation, and the demand for death with dignity pleads for the removal of these "unnatural" obstacles.

More generally, the demand for autonomy and the cry for dignity are asserted against a medicalization and institutionalization of the end of life that robs the old and the incurable of most of their autonomy and dignity: Intubated and electrified, with bizarre mechanical companions, confined and immobile, helpless and regimented, once proud and independent people find themselves cast in the role of passive, obedient, highly disciplined children. Death with dignity means, in the first instance, the removal of these added indignities and dehumanizations of the end of life.

One can only sympathize with this concern. Yet, even if successful, efforts to remove these obstacles would not yet produce a death with dignity. For one thing, not all obstacles to dignity are artificial and externally imposed. Infirmity and incompetence, dementia and immobility— all of them of natural origins—greatly limit human possibility, and for many of us they will be sooner or later unavoidable, the products of inevitable bodily or mental decay. Second, there is nothing of human dignity in the process of dying itself—only in the way we face it: At its best, death with complete dignity will always be compromised by the extinction of dignified humanity; it is, I suspect, a death-denying culture's anger about dying and mortality that expresses itself in the partly oxymoronic and unreasonable demand for dignity in death. Third, insofar as we seek better health and longer life, insofar as we turn to doctors to help us get better, we necessarily and voluntarily compromise our dignity: Being a patient rather than an agent is, humanly speaking, undignified. All people, especially the old, willingly, if unknowingly, accept a whole stable of indignities simply by seeking medical assistance. The really proud people refuse altogether to submit to doctors and hospitals. It is well to be reminded of these limits on our ability to roll back the indignities that assault the dying, so that we might acquire more realistic expectations about just how much dignity a "death with dignity" campaign can provide. Indeed, it is rather insensitive, not to say insulting, to imply that dignity will reign if only we can push back officious doctors, invasive machinery, litigation-shy hospital administrators, and the right-to-lifers and district attorneys of whom the administrators (and doctors) are afraid. The removal of impediments is not yet the creation of dignity.

A death with positive dignity—which may turn out to be something rare, even under the best of circumstances, like a life with dignity— entails more than the absence of external indignities. Dignity in the face of death cannot be given or conferred from the outside but requires a dignity of soul in the human being who faces it. This, despite the many claims to the contrary, neither the partisans of "death with dignity" nor the myriad servants of mankind, from the Department of Health and

Human Services to departments of medicine or psychiatry, can supply—though they can, perhaps, offer some assistance. The following distinction seems roughly apt: We might say that the *possibility* of a humanly dignified facing of death can be destroyed or undermined from without (and, of course, from within), but the *actualization* of that possibility depends largely on the soul, the character, the bearing of the dying man himself—i.e., on things *within*. To better understand the meaning of and prospects for death with dignity, we need first to think more about dignity itself, what it is.

Dignity is, to begin with, an undemocratic idea. The central notion, etymologically, both in English and in its Latin root (*dignitas*),[14] is that of worthiness, elevation, honor, nobility, height—in short, of excellence or virtue. In all its meanings it is a term of distinction; dignity is not something that, like a nose or a navel, is to be expected or found in every living human being. Dignity is, in principle, aristocratic.

It follows that dignity, thus understood, cannot be demanded or claimed; for it cannot be provided and it is not owed. One has no more *right* to dignity—and hence to dignity in death—than one has to beauty or courage or wisdom, desirable though these all may be.

One can, of course, seek to democratize the principle; one can argue that "excellence," "being worthy," is a property of all human beings, say, for example, in comparison with animals or plants, or with machines. This, I take it, is what is often meant by "*human* dignity." This is also what is implied when one asserts that much of the terminal treatment of dying patients is dehumanizing, or that attachments to catheters, respirators, and suction tubes hide the human countenance and thereby insult the dignity of the dying. This view is not without merit. Indeed, I myself earlier argued that the special dignity of the human species, thus understood, is the ground of the sanctity of human life. Yet on further examination this universal attribution of dignity to human beings pays tribute more to human potentiality, to the *possibilities* for human excellence. *Full* dignity, or dignity properly so called, would depend on the *realization* of these possibilities.

Moreover, to speak of dignity as predicable of all human beings, say, in contrast to animals, is, once again, to tie dignity to those distinctively human features of human animals, such as thought, image-making, the sense of beauty, freedom, friendship, and the moral life, and not the mere presence of life itself. *Among* human beings, there would still be, on any such material principle, distinctions to be made—unless one evacuates the meaning of the term, and the predicate "dignity" is held to add nothing to "born of woman." Thus if one were to accept, for example, Pascal's view that "Our whole dignity consists in thought" (by which he means, preeminently, self-consciousness and awareness of mortality), one would have to wonder about the relative ranking of those who think more and less, that is, who are more or less self-conscious. Or, if universal human dignity is grounded in the moral life, in that everyone faces and makes moral choices, *dignity* would seem to depend mainly on having a *good* moral life, that is, on choosing *well*. Clearly, we do not want to say that there is dignity—or much dignity—in the life of a paid killer, a slave-dealer, or a prostitute, or that they compare in dignity with Gandhi, Abraham Lincoln, or Joan of Arc. Is there not more dignity in the courageous than in the cowardly, in the moderate than in the self-indulgent, in the righteous than in the wicked?[15]

But courage, moderation, righteousness, and the other human virtues are not solely confined to the few. Many of us strive for them, with partial success, and still more of us do ourselves honor when we recognize and admire those people nobler and finer than ourselves. With proper models, proper rearing, and proper encouragement, many of us can be and act more in accord with our higher natures. In these ways, the openness to dignity can perhaps be democratized still further.

In truth, if we know how to look, we find evidence of human dignity all around us, in the valiant efforts ordinary people make to meet necessity, to combat adversity and disappointment, to provide for their children, to care for their parents, to help their neighbors, to serve their country. Life provides numerous hard occasions that call for endurance and equanimity, generosity and kindness, courage and self-command. Adversity sometimes brings out the best in a man, and often shows best what he is made of. Confronting our own death—or the deaths of our beloved ones—provides an opportunity for the exercise of our humanity, for the great and small alike. Death with dignity, in its most important sense, would mean a dignified attitude and virtuous conduct in the face of death.

What would such a dignified facing of death require? First of all, it would require knowing that one is dying. One cannot attempt to settle accounts, make arrangements, complete projects, keep promises, or say farewell if one does not know the score. Second, it requires that one remain to some degree an agent rather than (just) a patient. One cannot make a good end of one's life if one is buffeted about by forces beyond one's control, if one is denied a decisive share in decisions about medical treatments, institutionalization, and the way to spend one's remaining time. Third, it requires the upkeep—as much as possible—of one's familial, social, and professional relationships and activities. One cannot function as an actor if one has been swept off the stage and been abandoned by the rest of the cast. It would also seem to require some direct, self-conscious confrontation, in the loneliness of one's soul, with the brute fact and meaning of nearing one's end. Even, or especially, as he must be passive to the forces of decay, the dignified human being can preserve and reaffirm his humanity by seeing clearly and without illusion.[16] (It is for this reason, among others, that sudden and unexpected death, however painless, robs a man of the opportunity to have a dignified end.)

But as a dignified human life is not just a lonely project against an inevitable death, but a life whose meaning is entwined in human relationships, we must stress again the importance for a death with dignity—as for a life with dignity—of dignified human intercourse with all those around us. Who we are to ourselves is largely inseparable from who we are to and for others; thus, our own exercise of dignified humanity will depend crucially on continuing to receive respectful treatment from others. The manner in which we are addressed, what is said to us or in our presence, how our bodies are tended or our feelings regarded—in all these ways, our dignity in dying can be nourished and sustained. Dying people are all too easily reduced ahead of time to "thinghood" by those who cannot bear to deal with the suffering or disability of those they love. Objectification and detachment are understandable defenses. Yet this withdrawal of contact, affection, and care is probably the greatest single cause of the dehumanization of dying. Death with dignity requires absolutely that the survivors treat the human being at all times as if full god-like-ness remains, up to the very end.[17]

It will, I hope, now be perfectly clear that death with dignity, understood as living dignifiedly in the face of death, is not a matter of pulling plugs or taking poison. To speak this way—and it is unfortunately common to speak this way[18]—is to shrink still further the notion of human dignity, and thus heap still greater indignity upon the dying, beyond all the insults of illness and the medicalized bureaucratization of the end of life. If it is really death with dignity we are after, we must think in human and not technical terms. With these thoughts firmly in mind, we can turn in closing back to the matter of euthanasia.

EUTHANASIA: UNDIGNIFIED AND DANGEROUS

Having followed the argument to this point, even a friendly reader might chide me as follows: "Well and good to think humanistically, but tough practical dilemmas arise, precisely about the use of techniques, and they must be addressed. Not everyone is so fortunate as to be able to die at home, in the company of loving family, beyond the long reach of the medical—industrial complex. How should these technical decisions—about respirators and antibiotics and feeding tubes and, yes, even poison—be made, precisely in order to uphold human dignity and the sanctity of life that you say are so intermingled?" A fair question; I offer the following outline of an answer.

About treatment for the actually dying, there is in principle no difficulty. In my book, *Toward a More Natural Science,*[19] I have argued for the primacy of easing pain and suffering, along with supporting and comforting speech, and, more to the point, the need to draw back from some efforts at prolongation of life that prolong or increase only the patient's pain, discomfort, and suffering. Although I am mindful of the dangers and aware of the impossibility of writing explicit rules for ceasing treatment—hence the need for prudence—considerations of the individual's health, activity, and state of mind must enter into decisions of *whether* and *how vigorously* to treat if the decision is indeed to be for the patient's good. Ceasing treatment and allowing death to occur when (and if) it will can, under some circumstances, be quite compatible with the respect that life itself commands for itself. For life is to be revered not only as manifested in physiological powers, but also as these powers are organized in the form of *a* life, with its beginning, middle, and end. Or, in other words, life can be revered not only in its preservation, but also in the manner in which we allow a given life to reach its terminus.

What about so-called active euthanasia, the direct making dead of someone who is not yet dying or not dying "fast enough"? Elsewhere I have argued at great length against the practice of euthanasia *by physicians,* partly on the grounds of bad social consequences, but mainly on the grounds that killing patients—even those who ask for death—violates the inner meaning of the art of healing.[20] Powerful prudential arguments—unanswerable, in my view—have been advanced as to why legalized mercy-killing would be a disastrous social policy, at least for the United States. But some will insist that social policy cannot remain deaf to cries for human dignity, and that dangers must be run to preserve a dignified death through euthanasia, at least where it is requested. As our theme here is dignity and sanctity, I will confine my answer to the question of euthanasia and human dignity.

Let us begin with voluntary euthanasia—the request for assistance in dying. To repeat, the claim here is that the choice for death, because a free act, affirms the dignity of free will against dumb necessity. Or, using my earlier formulation, is it not precisely dignified for the "god-like" to put a voluntary end to the humiliation of that very godliness?

In response, let me start with the following questions. Do the people who are actually contemplating euthanasia *for themselves*—as opposed to their proxies who lead the euthanasia movement—generally put their requests in these terms? Or are they not rather looking for a way to end their troubles and pains? One can *sympathize* with such a motive, out of compassion, but can one admire it, out of respect? Is it really *dignified* to seek to escape from troubles for oneself? Is there, to repeat, not more dignity in courage than in its absence?

Euthanasia for one's own dignity is, at best, paradoxical, even self-contradictory: How can I honor myself by making myself nothing? Even if dignity were to consist solely in autonomy, is it not an embarrassment to claim that autonomy reaches its zenith precisely as it disappears? Voluntary euthanasia, in the name of *positive* dignity, does not make sense.

Acknowledging the paradox, some will still argue the cause of free-dom on a more narrow ground: The prospect of euthanasia increases human freedom by increasing options. It is, of course, a long theoretical question whether human freedom is best understood—and best served—through the increase of possibilities. But as a practical matter, in the *present* case, I am certain that this view is mistaken. On the contrary, the opening up of this "option" of assisted suicide will greatly constrain human choice. For the choice for death is not one option among many, but an option to end all options. Socially, there will be great social pressure on the aged and the vulnerable to exercise this option. Once there looms the legal alternative of euthanasia, it will plague and burden every decision made by any seriously ill, elderly person—not to speak of their more powerful caretakers—even without the subtle hints and pressures applied to them by others.[21]

And, thinking about others, is it dignified to ask or demand that someone else become my killer? It may be sad that one is unable to end one's own life, but can it conduce to either party's dignity to make the request? Consider its double meaning if made to a son or daughter: Do you love me so little as to force me to live on? Do you love me so little as to want me dead? What person in full possession of their own dignity would inflict such a duty on anyone they loved?

What, indeed, does human dignity require of us, regarding our loved ones, as we grow old, decline, and die? I have thought much about this question. Arguing now against myself, I confess that I look ahead with deep horror on the prospect that I might fall into a protracted state of such reduced humanity—say, with loss of memory, self-control, and the ability sensibly to converse—that I become a burden or even an object of loathing for my spouse and children. Under such conditions, it has often seemed to me that it would be better—indeed, nobler and more digni-fied—for me to take my own life than to live so as to cause my children to harden their hearts or to harbor secret wishes for my death—a horror to be prevented not for me but *for them*. It is hard to imagine anything worse, parentally speaking, than for a parent *by his very existence* to force a child's heart to turn against him. Suicide for such "altruistic" reasons, unlike suicide to escape from my own pain, would not appear to be base or undignified; it seems to belong, at first glance, in the category of noble self-sacrifice. But there is a catch: To be in fact noble, my suicide would have to be accomplished in full secrecy—no mean feat for the demented and immobile; no suicide *known* to be a suicide bequeaths anything but pain and guilt to his loved ones—the very thing that I would be trying to avoid. But suppose, now, that euthanasia (assisted suicide) were legal: My children—everyone—would be invited to deliberate about, wish for, encourage, and even participate in the death (and killing) of those they love. What a legacy! The very thing I have imagined committing suicide to prevent, the new dispensation will necessarily have brought into being. Can this really be death with dignity?

Of course, the whole thing could be made impersonal. No requests to family members, only to physicians. But precisely the same point applies: How can one demand care and humanity from one's physician, and, at the same time, demand that he play the role of technical dispenser of death? To turn the matter over to nonphysicians, that is, to technically competent professional euthanizers, is, of course, to completely dehumanize the matter.[22]

Proponents of euthanasia do not understand human dignity, which, at best, they confuse with humaneness. One of their favorite arguments proves this point: Why, they say, do we put animals out of their misery but insist on compelling fellow human beings to suffer to the bitter end? Why, if it is not a contradiction for the veterinarian, does the medical ethic absolutely rule out mercy killing? Is this not simply inhumane?

Perhaps inhumane, but not thereby inhuman. On the contrary, it is precisely because animals are not human that we must treat them (merely) humanely. We put dumb animals to sleep because they do not know that they are dying, because they can make nothing of their misery or mortality, and therefore, because they cannot live deliberately—i.e., humanly—in the face of their own suffering or dying. They cannot live out a fitting end. Compassion for their weakness and dumbness is our only appropriate emotion, and given our responsibility for their care and well-being, we do the only humane thing we can. But when a conscious human being asks us for death, by that very action he displays the presence of something that precludes our regarding him as a dumb animal. Humanity is owed humanity, not humaneness. Humanity is owed the bolstering of the human, even or especially in its dying moments, in resistance to the temptation to ignore its presence in the sight of suffering.

What humanity needs most in the face of evils is courage, the ability to stand against fear and pain and thoughts of nothingness. The deaths we most admire are those of people who, knowing that they are dying, face the fact frontally and act accordingly: They set their affairs in order; they arrange what could be final meetings with their loved ones, and yet, with strength of soul and a small reservoir of hope, they continue to live and work and love as much as they can for as long as they can. Because such conclusions of life require courage, they call for our encouragement—and for the many small speeches and deeds that shore up the human spirit against despair and defeat.

And what of nonvoluntary euthanasia, for those too disabled to request it for themselves—the comatose, the senile, the psychotic: Can this be said to be in the service of *their* human dignity? If dignity is, as the autonomy people say, tied crucially to consciousness and will, nonvoluntary or "proxy-voluntary" euthanasia can never be a dignified act for the one euthanized. On their own view, the situation is beneath dignity. Indeed, it is precisely the absence of dignified humanity that invites the thought of active euthanasia in the first place.

Is it really true that such people are beneath all human dignity? I suppose it depends on the particulars. Many people in greatly reduced states still retain clear, even if partial, participation in human relations. They may respond to kind words or familiar music; they may keep up pride in their appearance or in the achievements of the grandchildren; they may take pleasure in reminiscences or simply in having someone who cares enough to be present; conversely, they may be irritated or hurt or sad, even appropriately so; and, even nearer bottom, they may be able to return a smile or a glance in response to a drink of water or a change of bedding or a bath. Because we really do not know their inner life—what they feel and understand—we run the risk of robbing them of opportunities for dignity by treating them as if they had none. It does not follow from the fact that *we* would never willingly trade places with them that *they* have *nothing* left worth respecting.

But what, finally, about the very bottom of the line, say, people in a "persistent vegetative state," unresponsive, contorted, with no evident ability to interact with the environment? What human dignity remains here? Why should we not treat such human beings as we (properly) treat dumb animals, and put them out of "their misery"[23]? I grant that one faces here the hardest case for the argument I am advancing. Yet, one probably cannot be absolutely sure, even here, about the complete absence of inner life or awareness of their surroundings. In some cases, admittedly extremely rare, persons recover from profound coma (even with flat EEG); and they sometimes report having had partial yet vivid awareness of what was said and done to them, though they had given no external evidence of same. But beyond any restraint owing to ignorance, I would also myself be restrained by the human form, by *human blood*, and by what I owe to the full human life that this particular instance of humanity once lived. I would gladly stand aside and let die, say in the advent of pneumonia; I would do little beyond the minimum to sustain life; but I would not countenance the giving of lethal injections or the taking of other actions deliberately intending the patient's death. Between only undignified courses of action, this strikes me as the least undignified—especially for myself.

I have no illusions that it is easy to live with a Karen Ann Quinlan or a Nancy Cruzan or the baby Linares. I think I sufficiently appreciate the anguish of their parents or their children, and the distortion of their lives and the lives of their families. I also know that, when hearts break and people can stand it no longer, mercy-killing will happen, and I think we should be prepared to excuse it—as we generally do—when it occurs in this way. But an excuse is not yet a justification, and very far from dignity.

What then should we conclude, as a matter of social policy? We should reject the counsel of those who, seeking to drive a wedge between human dignity and the sanctity of life, argue the need for active euthanasia, especially in the name of death with dignity. For it is precisely the setting of fixed limits on violating human life that makes possible our efforts at dignified relations with our fellow-men, especially when their neediness and disability try our patience. We will never be able to relate even decently to people if we are entitled always to consider that one option before us is to make them dead. Thus, when the advocates for euthanasia press us with the most heart-rending cases, we should be sympathetic but firm. Our response should be neither "Yes, for mercy's sake" nor "Murder! Unthinkable!" but "Sorry. No." Above all, we must not allow ourselves to become self-deceived: We must never seek to relieve *our own* frustrations and bitterness over the lingering deaths of others by pretending that we can kill them to sustain *their dignity.*

CODA

The ancient Greeks knew about hybris and its tragic fate. We modern rationalists do not. We do not yet understand that the project for the conquest of death leads only to dehumanization, that any attempt to gain the tree of life by means of the tree of knowledge leads inevitably also to the hemlock, and that the utter rationalization of life under the banner of the will gives rise to a world in which the victors live long enough to finish life demented and without choice. The human curse is to discover only too late the evils latent in acquiring the goods we wish for.

Against the background of enormous medical success, terminal illness and incurable disease appear as failures and as affronts to human pride. We refuse to be caught resourceless. Thus, having adopted a largely technical approach to human life and having medicalized so much of the end of life, we now are willing to contemplate a final technical solution for the evil of human finitude and for our own technical (but unavoidable) "failure," as well as for the degradations of life that are the unintended consequences of our technical successes. This is dangerous folly. People who care for autonomy and human dignity should try rather to reverse this dehumanization of the last stages of life, instead of giving dehumanization its final triumph by welcoming the desperate goodbye-to-all-that contained in one final plea for poison.

The present crisis that leads some to press for active euthanasia is really an opportunity to learn the limits of the medicalization of life and death and to recover an appreciation of living with and against mortality. It is an opportunity to remember and affirm that there remains a residual human wholeness—however precarious—that can be cared for even in the face of incurable and terminal illness. Should we cave in, should we choose to become technical dispensers of death, we will not only be abandoning our loved ones and our duty to care; we will exacerbate the worst tendencies of modern life, embracing technicism and so-called humaneness where encouragement and humanity are both required and sorely lacking. On the other hand, should we hold fast, should we decline the principle of autonomy and its deadly options, should we learn that finitude is no disgrace and that dignity can be cared for to the very end, we may yet be able to stem the rising tide that threatens permanently to submerge the best hopes for human dignity.

NOTES AND REFERENCES

1. Herodotus *Histories*, 1: 30–33.

2. Precisely such a (constitutionally protected) right to die (i.e., to become dead), claimed by proxies on behalf of a permanently comatose other, was asserted in the *Cruzan* case, the first such case to be decided by the United States Supreme Court. See *Cruzan by Cruzan* v. *Director, Missouri Department of Health* 110 S. Ct. 2841 (1990). The court refused in this instance to grant the family's request for removal of nutrition and hydration, primarily because it held there was insufficient evidence about Nancy Cruzan's own wishes. Though the majority opinion struggled to avoid speaking, in its own name, of a "right to die," it

did assume, "for purposes of this case, . . . that the United States Constitution would grant a competent person a constitutionally protected right to refuse lifesaving hydration and nutrition" (p. 2852). (This suggestion relied on an analysis of "liberty interests" under the Due Process Clause of the Fourteenth Amendment.) While admittedly not yet the clear enunciation of a constitutional "right to die," the slide down the slippery slope accelerates. Far better in my view is Justice Scalia's concurring opinion, which argues persuasively that, according to our constitutional traditions, "the power of the State to prohibit suicide is unquestionable":

> What I have said above is not meant to suggest that I would think it desirable, if we were sure that Nancy Cruzan wanted to die, to keep her alive by the means at issue here. I only assert that the Constitution has nothing to say about the subject. To raise up a constitutional right here we would have to create out of nothing (for it exists neither in text nor tradition) some constitutional principle whereby, although the State may insist that an individual come in out of the cold and eat food, it may not insist that he take medicine; and although it may pump his stomach empty of poison he has ingested, it may not fill his stomach with food he has failed to ingest. (p. 2863)

For a fine critique of efforts to establish a right to die, see Hadley Arkes, "When Bungling Practice Is Joined to Absurd Theory: Doctors, Philosophers, and the Right to Die," *The World & I* (September 1990): 599–615.

3.   Indeed, the title first proposed to me by the conveners of the conference was "Death with Dignity *versus* the Sanctity of Life."

4.   Some people, in contrast, are delighted with this polarized framing of the question, for they see it as the conflict between a vigorous humanism and an anachronistic otherworldliness, foisted on the West by the Judeo-Christian tradition. For those who deny the sacred, it is desirable to represent the arguments against suicide or mercy-killing (or abortion) as purely religious in character— there being in truth, on their view, nothing higher than human dignity. The chief proponent of the recent "Humane and Dignified Death Initiative" in California is reported to have said that he was seeking to "overturn the sanctity of life principle" in American law. See Robert Risley, quoted in Richard Doerflinger, "Pulling the Plug," *Columbia* (August 1988): 13–15, at 13.

5.   Baruch A. Brody, "A Historical Introduction to Jewish Casuistry on Suicide and Euthanasia," in *Suicide and Euthanasia*, Baruch A. Brody, ed. (Dordrecht, Netherlands: Kluwer Academic Publishers, 1989), 39–75, at 39.

6.   The Babylonian Talmud, Tractate Sanhedrin, fol. 74a. [A complete English translation of talmudic references is available in *The Babylonian Talmud*, R. Isidore Epstein, ed. (London: Soncino Press, 1969)—Ed.] See also the discussion of this issue in Immanuel Jakobovits, *Jewish Medical Ethics* (New York: Bloch Publishing Co., 1959), 53–58.

7.   This is, of course, as it should be. The most important insights on which decent society rests—e.g., the taboos against incest, cannibalism, murder, and adultery—are too important to be imperiled by reason's poor power to give them a convincing defense. Such taboos might themselves be the incarnation of

reason, even as they resist attempts to give them logical demonstration; like the axioms of geometry, they might be at once incapable of proof and yet not in need of proof, i.e., self-evident to anyone not morally blind. What follows, then, is more a search for insight than an attempt at proof.

8. Nonreligious readers will, no doubt, express suspicion at my appeal to a biblical text for what I will claim is a universal or philosophical explanation of the taboo against murder. This suspicion will be further increased by the content of the text cited. Nevertheless, properly interpreted, I believe the teaching of the passage stands free of its especially biblical roots and offers a profound insight into the ground of our respect for human life. Indeed, great thinkers, such as Rousseau and Kant, have read the book of *Genesis* philosophically and drawn on it for similar arguments. To treat this depository of wisdom as "religious" (or "metaphysical"), and hence as purely sectarian, is pure thoughtlessness. Let the critics forgo their prejudices and try to show that the arguments or the insights are defective.

9. This respect for human life, and the self-conscious establishment of society on this premise, separates human beings from the rest of the animals. This separation is made emphatic by the institution of meat-eating (*Genesis* 9:1–4), permitted to man here for the first time. (One can, I believe, show that the permission to eat meat is a concession to human blood-lust and voracity, not something cheerfully and happily endorsed.) Yet, curiously, even animal life must be treated with respect. The blood, which is identified as the life, cannot be eaten. Human life, as we shall see more clearly, is thus both continuous and discontinuous with animal life.

10. The second part of verse 6 seems to make two points: Man is in the image of God (i.e., god-*like*), and man was *made* thus by God. The decisive point is the first. Man's creatureliness cannot be the reason for avoiding bloodshed; the animals too were made by God, yet permission to kill them for food has just been given. The full weight rests on man's *being* "in the image of God."

11. Fittingly, this assertion *about* man is here made *to man*, only at the point when men, by themselves, undertake to rise above their animal condition, i.e., when they quit the state of nature and take up the state of right. The previous biblical remarks about man's god-likeness were made by God but not addressed to human hearers (except for us readers).

12. In the first creation story, *Genesis* 1–2:3, man is created straightaway in God's likeness; in this second account, man is, to begin with, made of dust, and he *acquires* god-like qualities only at the end, and then only in transgressing.

13. Does this mean that those who murder forfeit their claim to be humanly respected because they implicitly have denied the humanity of their victim (and, thus, in principle, of their own—and all other—human life)? In other words, do men need to act in accordance with the self-knowledge of human godliness in order to be treated accordingly? Or, conversely, do we rather respect the humanity of murderers when we punish them, even capitally, treating them not as crazed or bestial but as responsible moral agents, who accept the fair consequences of their deeds? Or is the capitalness of the punishment not a theoretical matter, but a practical one, intended mainly to deter by fear those whose self-love or will-to-power will not listen to reason? These are vexed questions, too

complicated to sort out quickly, and, in any case, beyond the point of the present discussion. Yet the relevant difficulty persists.

14.   The English word "dignity" derives from the Latin *dignitas*, which, according to the *White and Riddle Latin-English Dictionary*, means (1) a being worthy, worthiness, merit, desert, (2) dignity, greatness, grandeur, authority, rank, and (3) (of inanimate things) worth, value, excellence. The noun is cognate with the adjective *dignus* (the root *DIC*, related to the Sanskrit *DIC* and the Greek *DEIK*, means "to bring to light," "to show," "to point out"), literally "pointed out" or "shown" and hence "worthy" or "deserving" (of persons), and "suitable," "fitting," "becoming," or "proper" (of things).

"Dignity," in the *Oxford English Dictionary*, is said to have eight meanings, the four relevant ones I reproduce here: (1) The quality of being worthy or honourable; worthiness, worth, nobleness, excellence (for instance, "The real dignity of a man lies not in what he *has*, but in what he *is*," or "The dignity of this act was worth the audience of kings"); (2) Honourable or high estate, position, or estimation; honour, degrees of estimation, rank (for instance, "Stones, though in dignitie of nature inferior to plants," or "Clay and clay differs in dignity, whose dust is both alike"); (3) An honourable office, rank, or title; a high official or titular position (for instance, "He . . . distributed the civil and military dignities among his favorites and followers"); (4) Nobility or befitting elevation of aspect, manner, or style; becoming or fit stateliness, gravity (for instance, "A dignity of dress adorns the Great").

15.   This is not necessarily to say that one should treat other people, including those who eschew dignity, as if they lacked it. This is a separable question. It may be salutary to treat people on the basis of their capacities to live humanly, despite even great falling short or even willful self-degradation. Yet this would, in the moral sphere at least, require what we expect and demand of people that they behave worthily and that we hold them responsible for their own conduct.

16.   The Homeric warriors, preoccupied with mortality and refusing to hide away in a corner waiting for death to catch them unawares, went boldly forward to meet it, armed only with their own prowess and large hearts; in facing death frontally, in the person of another similarly self-conscious hero, they wrested a human victory over blind necessity, even in defeat. On a much humbler scale, the same opportunity is open to anyone willing to look death in the face.

17.   An earlier version of this essay elicited the following thoughtful comment from a wise New York attorney, John F. Cannon, supplementing (critically) my analysis of dignity yet strongly supporting this conclusion and my argument about euthanasia that follows from it:

> I take "dignity's" reference to be not merely to something that is "in" a person, but also, perhaps primarily, to the affective response that is "fitting" (*dignus*) for others to make to what is "in" the person. The notion that one *has* "dignity," or *is* "dignified," involves only part of this broader meaning: it suggests that what a person is, ontologically or morally, entitles him to be regarded and treated with dignity by his fellow man. In this incomplete sense of the word, a person can be said to "have" dignity whether or not anyone else is aware of his existence or actions. If a person who is dying has ceased to be an agent and has been "attached to

catheters, respirators, and suction tubes [that] hide the human countenance" or has "been swept off the stage and been abandoned by the rest of the cast," he can still respond virtuously to his awful predicament (in the former case, only if he is aware of it), and if he so responds, he can be said to have "lost" his dignity only in the sense that others have refused to grant it to him. He is no less "worthy" a person, but what he is "worthy of" has been withheld, or worse. Dignity, in other words, is something that is simultaneously earned and conferred.

From this perspective, to argue that assisted suicide or active euthanasia is a means to the end of "death with dignity" is to make the absurd claim that if I cannot maintain a "dignified attitude and conduct in the face of [my own] death," or if I manage to do that but it turns out to be too much to ask others to accord me the dignity my virtuous conduct deserves, killing me is somehow a way to let me die *with my dignity*; in the case of a loved one who is dying, it is to claim that if he is hopelessly racked by fear, pain and self-pity, or if the degree of courage he shows in the face of death merits more compassion and affection for him that I can bear to give, his *dignity*, and mine, will somehow be advanced by killing him.

18. A perfect instance is the recent California Initiative. It proposed amending the name of the existing California statute from "Natural Death Act" to "Humane and Dignified Death Act," but its only substantive change was to declare and provide for "the right of the terminally ill to voluntary, humane, and *dignified* doctor-assisted *aid in dying*," "aid in dying" meaning "any medical procedure that would terminate the life of the qualified patient swiftly, painlessly, and humanely." A (merely) natural death is to be made "dignified" simply by having it deliberately produced by (dignified) doctors.

19. Leon R. Kass, *Toward a More Natural Science: Biology and Human Affairs* (New York: The Free Press, 1985). See, especially chapters 7 and 8.

20. Leon R. Kass, "Neither for Love nor Money: Why Physicians Must Not Kill," *The Public Interest* (Winter 1989): 25–46.

21. For a superb discussion of this and other dangers see Yale Kamisar, "Some Non-Religious Views Against Proposed 'Mercy-Killing' Legislation," *Minnesota Law Review* 42 (May 1958): 969–1042. Reprinted, with a new preface by Professor Kamisar, in "The Slide Toward Mercy-Killing," *Child and Family Reprint Booklet Series*, 1987.

22. For a chilling picture of a fully rationalized and technically managed death, see the account of the Park Lane Hospital for the Dying in Aldous Huxley's *Brave New World*.

23. Once again we should be careful about our speech. It may be a great source of misery for *us* to see them in this state, but it is not at all clear that *they* *feel* or *have* misery. Precisely the ground for considering them beneath the human threshold is that nothing registers with them. This point is relevant to the "termination-of-feeding" cases, in which it is argued (in self-contradiction) that death by starvation is both humane and not in these instances cruel: Someone who is too far gone to suffer from a death by starvation is, to begin with, not suffering at all.

8

Good Rules Have Good Reasons: A Response to Leon Kass

Ronald M. Green

I find Leon Kass's remarks deeply moving. At many points they display a quality of moral wisdom rare in so much contemporary ethical discourse. I also substantially share many of Kass's convictions and concerns, and I am led to many similar practical conclusions in regard to many aspects of our treatment of the dying. For example, I strongly agree that dignity in death, as in life, is not so much a matter of the vicissitudes to which one is exposed as it is of the way one responds to them. I agree that the principal focus of our efforts with respect to the dying must be on proper care in order to create the appropriately human circumstances for dying rather than simply expediting the dying process. With Kass, I fear the coercion likely to be brought to bear on elderly and dying patients by a culture of euthanasia, one that "expects" a voluntary death on the part of those who have become emotional or financial burdens.[1] I also share Kass's concern for the emotional and practical distortions in our relationship to the dying that are likely to be induced when care becomes confused with killing. Above all, I share his fears about the impact on medical professionals of the mentality that sees killing as a part of the medical armamentarium. As a Jew, I have a special concern in this area. The writings of Robert J. Lifton and others have shown us how slippery is the slope that lies between any form of medically authorized killing and mass murder.[2] In my role as a teacher of ethics, I frequently find myself uttering to students the old adage, *abusus non tollit usus*—a practice's potential for abuse does not necessarily mean it must be prohibited. But here, I believe, the experiment has already been run, and we have learned enough from the ghastly record of our century to understand why any empowerment of medical professionals to kill is undertaken at the gravest peril.[3]

Despite these important areas of agreement, I am uncomfortable with the mode of argumentation in Professor Kass's paper. My disagreements begin at the theoretical level but lead to several important differences in practical result. Since I want to make this a productive exchange, I shall go out of my way to accentuate these differences—to the point, perhaps, of making them sharper than they are. In the end, we shall see, my theoretical preferences render me more willing than Kass to develop some responses to urgent problems at the end of life that have been partly created by medicine's limitless ability to intrude on the dying process.

My disagreements with Kass begin with his effort to establish a basis for the sanctity of human life that somehow transcends human willing. In the course of his discussion of why murder is morally wrong, Kass observes that our basic prohibition against homicide can partly be explained in terms of the value that each person places on his or her life. In these terms, says Kass, "murder is wrong because it opposes this will-to-live, because it deprives another of life against his will, because it kills someone who does not want to die (and who has not committed some offense that might justify ignoring his will to live)." Kass goes on to say that "This sort of reason would explain why suicide—willed self-killing—could be right, while murder—killing an innocent person against his will—would always be wrong" (p. 124).

Nevertheless, Kass continues, "There is something obviously troublesome about this way of thinking about crimes against persons." This is because "the most abominable practices, proscribed in virtually all societies," including such practices as consensual murder, incest or slavery, "are not excused by consent." This suggests to Kass that the violence and evil done to another are independent of the state of the will of the individual involved. Instead, he contends, it resides in the intrinsic dignity of a human life. As his argument proceeds, Kass traces this dignity, in quasireligious terms, to each human being's "divine-like status," (p. 127) to our formation, in both spiritual and physical terms, in God's image. Kass senses some difficulties in this mode of reasoning. If human beings are sacred entities, how can we explain the permission in the same biblical sources that establish this sanctity for the taking of the life of one who has killed another? Do purely practical and pragmatic needs explain this exception to the prohibition on killing? But if so, where does such pragmatism end? Are complex retributive notions at work whereby those who kill another are thought to forfeit their sacred protectability? Or, by their submission to punishment, are such condemned persons conceived as retaining and expressing a purely moral dimension of sanctity that transcends bodily welfare? In different ways, each of these latter solutions disturbs Kass's unitary solution to the problem of sanctity because they reintroduce an element of volition or social need into the calculus or because they subordinate physical existence to spiritual claims.

These conceptual complexities should suggest to us that something may have gone wrong in the reasoning process that leads Kass to his understanding of the concept of human sanctity. And, indeed, I think we can see that the problem begins with a false dichotomy. In Kass's thinking, there are only two alternatives. "Is the life of another human being to be respected," he asks, "only because that person (or society) *deems* or *wills* it respectable, or is it to be respected because *it is in itself* respectable?" (p. 125). Since the nearly universal prohibitions against forms of consensual coercion suggest that the former is not an adequate way to understand our moral thinking in this area, the only alternative, Kass concludes, is to find and develop an intrinsic basis for the sanctity of human life, a basis somehow independent of "the needs of society or the will of the victim" (p. 129). This basis might involve some axiomatic fundamental norm "incapable of proof" and "yet not in need of proof," something "self-evident to anyone not morally blind" (p. 143, n.7).

What Kass fails to consider, however, is that there is another explanation for these universal prohibitions on consensual killing or coercion, one that is intermediate between the view tracing all norms to the volition of the person at stake and the one deriving them from an inherent sanctity unrelated to reasoned human willing and not amenable to further rational analysis. This intermediate explanation recognizes that rational persons bent on pursuing their individual ends would nevertheless sometimes find it rational to place limits on the sovereignty of their wills. Historically, a good illustration of this is to be found in the prohibition on dueling. Recognizing the powerfully coercive forces of honor and reputation that can bear down on the individual and the destructive cycle of violence that can result, civilized societies have almost universally elaborated a series of prohibitions in this area. These prohibitions disallow individual willing in this area, but they are by no means unrelated to individual freedom of willing or to the rational interests of persons. To borrow a phrase from Garrett Hardin, we might say that these prohibitions involve the exercise of "mutual coercion mutually agreed on."[4]

It is not hard to see that similar processes of reasoning underlie the series of prohibitions arrayed by civilized societies against consensual murder, incest, and the like. All agreements in these areas have come to be recognized by legal systems as involving what are called "unconscionable contracts." We prohibit consensual incest, for example, in part because we have recognized that the subtle power relations involved prevent us from distinguishing between an instance of consensual incest, even if it were to exist, and one in which coercion is involved. The same is true where slavery and murder are concerned. In the case of murder there is the additional sobering consideration that the victims of allegedly consensual killing will not usually be around to challenge or dispute their killer's legal defense.

All these perfectly rational considerations help explain these prohibitions without resort to claims about the irreducibly wrongful or self-evidently wicked nature of the conduct involved. The same processes of reasoning, I might add, also explain the valid exceptions to the sanctity of life elaborated in the areas of punishment, war, and the like. Here exceptions must be made if personal security is to be preserved, and no rhetoric about "life's sanctity" has prevailed against this moral common sense. In sum, we do not have to yield our moral thinking in this area, as Kass seems to do, to the opaque and murky realm of self-evident norms or religious appeals. This whole normative area is not impenetrable to human reason or to a view that founds ethics on a full conception of rational human willing.

So much for theoretical issues. Let us now return to the questions before us and, in particular, to the complex matter of euthanasia. We will see that because of this theoretical disagreement, I will be led in my thinking to some important differences in practical conclusion from Kass.

We can begin by observing that deriving human moral norms from rational willing does not, in this area, any more than in those just touched on, require that a person's willing always be respected and that voluntary euthanasia, understood as the active killing of a terminally ill or suffering patient with his or her consent, should be allowed. The key question to be answered is not what some particular individuals at some time might happen to want done to them, but what rational members of a social order concerned over the longer term to best protect their own freedom and autonomy would find it rational to permit.

When we put the question this way, many of the traditional objections to active euthanasia, some of which are sensitively developed by Kass, make a reappearance. Fears of abuse, so well founded both in logic and experience, mass before us. The subtle and not-so-subtle forms of coercion imposed on the dying or on those patients merely "in the way" form a pressing concern. The potentially dramatic alteration in our attitudes toward the dying must be factored into our thinking, as must our changed attitudes toward the medical profession (and that profession's understanding of itself). On the side of medical necessity, it must also be asked whether a transformation of traditional attitudes and practices is really even needed. A sensitive application of more traditional norms permitting cessation of therapy or the "caring" use of analgesia allow us to cope with many of the hard cases we face today. Changes in attitude can also play a role. Particularly important is Kass's wise reminder that human dignity is bound up above all not in what we suffer but how we respond, as individuals and communities, to that suffering.

All these considerations suggest to me, as they do to Kass, that we must be very reluctant to authorize active euthanasia in any form. Wherein, then, do I disagree with him? What, on balance, is the practical import of our difference in theoretical approaches, between my tracing of norms to intelligently and sensitively exercised rational willing versus his employment of a religiously supported emphasis on the inherent sanctity of life?

I have two answers to this question. First, it seems to me that a focus on informed willing might open up the possibility of a more refined consideration of our conduct in the difficult marginal area that exists between active and passive measures. Behind the prohibition on active euthanasia lies a valid, reasoned fear we have of ever authorizing individuals to kill. But these concerns need not extend to the permission for withholding care, even forms of care now commonly expected in medical settings. I realize that the intention to end a life can be the same whether we actively kill or withhold an available therapy. But the rightness or wrongness of deeds is not measured solely by intention. Above all, we must consider the import of the practical rule we elaborate whenever we justify a form of conduct. Considered in this light, however, there is a world of difference between any form of cessation of therapy and any form of killing. Particularly important here are the implications of these two practices in cases of error or abuse. A physician or nurse who abuses a right to kill is a lethal agent who can destroy many persons including those who challenge their deeds. In contrast, a doctor or nurse who withholds care, whether it be resuscitation, normal antibiotics, or even food and fluids, does damage that by its nature will ordinarily be limited to the infirm patients in their care whose difficulties stem from a preexisting illness. I do not wish to underestimate the possibilities for harm here: A nursing home supervisor who fails to provide basic care to his or her geriatric patients is a social threat. But we can see the point I am making by comparing this kind of individual with the physician, nurse, or nurse's aid in this setting who carries a lethal syringe and who believes that it is permissible to kill patients "to end their suffering."

On the other side of this matter, medical technology has also created urgent new reasons for rethinking the norms in this area. Since patients can be artificially sustained in so many new ways today, there is good reason for addressing a problem that medicine itself has created. Unlike

Kass, I am not convinced that a decision to die, the choice to "cease being a choosing being," is patently absurd or irrational. Life involves many choices that have the effect of foreclosing future choices of the same kind, and the choice of death or a course leading to death is only the most extreme of these. But we do not ordinarily prohibit persons from making many such momentous decisions. There are also many good reasons why rational persons would wish to escape life and be free of the ministrations of the medical system. Extreme suffering, personal despair, and even the wish to preserve one's "dignity"—in the limited but valid sense of wishing to retain control over one's body and one's fate—can all be valid reasonings for wanting to die. Kass acknowledges that a "humanly dignified facing of death can be destroyed or undermined from without," and he perceives that it is an entirely natural usage of the term "indignity" to apply it to "intubated and electrified" patients "cast in the roles of . . . children" (p. 132). But in his effort to stress the importance of interior attitudes as the measure of dignity, he minimizes the seriousness of these external intrusions on the dying process. We must not forget, however, that for some persons "dignity" does have the meaning of not spending their last days being treated like an infant or a noisome inanimate object, or of not being subjected to conditions that disempower them and alter their personality so as to render them unrecognizable to their loved ones.

These considerations suggest to me the need for some creative re-thinking of the meaning of cessation of care in various settings. How would my thinking compare here with Kass's? I am not entirely sure, since he barely addresses this question in his paper. I suspect, however, that what he says about the sanctity of life, about the care owed those who are sick or dying, and about the priority of courage in the face of suffering would lead him to be less concerned than I am about the brute suffering and social or emotional burdens medicine has helped create. In my view, this may be an instance where a thinker is likely to be "be-witched" by his own impassioned language in ways that lead him to lose sight of the basic rational concerns we need to address in this area. For my part, almost anything that is construable under the rubric of "cessa-tion of care" might be acceptable, when such cessation is voluntarily requested by the patient or by appropriate patient proxies. This would certainly include cessation of food and fluids for vegetative or terminal patients and for patients of any age for whom choosing to die would be a rational alternative. I realize that this extreme position trespasses on some of the ground Kass has staked out for us. Practices such as those I favor can certainly engender attitudes toward the dying that we all might eventually regard as pernicious. But I reiterate my belief that limitations in this area are principally explained in terms of the constraints rational persons would choose to impose on themselves. Those constraints, I believe, are clearest where active killing is involved and become both correspondingly less clear and more intrusive where such killing is not involved.

A second area in which I believe the approach I am commending might lead me to different practical conclusions than Kass has to do with the matter of "assisted suicide." I note that Kass is very clear about the problems created by asking physicians to play a role in the killing of patients. But in this paper he never pauses to consider whether there might be a place for new social forms that would enhance individuals' own ability to end their suffering or to bring life to a conclusion more in keeping with their own wishes and desires. An example of this was recently provided in the Rosier case in Florida, where Mrs. Rosier, facing the painful end of a long bout with cancer, was given by her physician husband the sleeping pills she attempted to use to end her life in the manner she preferred. Not long ago, a similar episode occurred in my own family. A relative, an attractive and active woman in her mid-sixties who had nursed her own elderly father until his death following more than a decade of suffering from Alzheimer's disease, chose to end her own life after she learned that she had entered the early stages of the same illness.

In these and similar cases, physicians may help supply the means by which these individuals seek to end their own lives. In these cases, physicians are not killers, but neither can they be described as merely withholding therapy. Their conduct might be described as somehow intermediate between these two or, more properly I think, as involving steps taken to clear socially imposed obstacles to individual autonomy (in this case the prescription process). In the complex analysis of this option, I am frankly not clear about the final position I would want to hold. With Kass, I fear the easy route opened up here to medical neglect, and I deeply fear the subtle or not-so-subtle forms of pressure that might be applied to individuals to convince them "heroically" or "courageously" to end their own lives. In our culture, we surely do not need talk of any "duty to die."[5]

At the same time, for all these fears, I am not persuaded that rational persons would necessarily prohibit all forms of assisted suicide in view of the fine balance that must be struck between our need for mutual protection, on the one hand, and, on the other, our sometimes equally urgent need to procure relief from suffering and to retain control of our destiny at the end of life. Unlike Kass, I am not entirely convinced that human dignity is not sometimes compromised by forms of illness that lead to a progressive loss of personal control. I concede that dignity has many meanings, but the desire to determine the course of one's own life is certainly a part of what we mean by expressing or exercising our dignity, and Kass's language should not lead him entirely to neglect this dimension of the concept. Nor should we, as rational persons, ignore the needs of those who conceive of their dignity as involving some control in such circumstances.

Perhaps the fitting solution to this difficult problem is one inadvertently suggested by Kass himself (p. 140). We can uphold the social prohibition on assisted suicide while legally "excusing" the conduct of physicians or family members who employ this resort for valid reasons. But if we choose to select this course, let us not deceive ourselves. Whether we acknowledge it or not, an active process of moral reasoning underlies this strategy. It is not merely that we think something wrong but excuse it. Rather, in failing to punish, we make the judgment that in a specific instance a form of conduct was not altogether wrong and may even have been morally right.

In this commentary on Kass's thoughtful paper, I have tried to sketch this process of reasoning and the pattern of justification that underlies concrete judgments of this sort. The approach I am arguing for does not appeal to self-evidence nor make use of religious arguments beyond human rational willing to justify the norms we uphold. It recognizes instead that it is in all our interests sometimes to impose restraints on one another to preserve our reasoned capacity to pursue our ends. The key questions in medical care at the end of life, I remain convinced, are precisely when such restraints make sense and when they do not. I believe that by thinking rationally about these matters, by avoiding seductive appeals to self-evidence, to persuasive definitions or to morally opaque intuitions, whether of a religious or secular sort, we can best achieve the kind of clarity these issues demand.

In the end, I must say, for all my agreement with many of the concrete points he makes in this paper, I differ with Kass over matters of moral methodology, and, in relation to this, over what we regard to be the important moral threats facing our civilization. He perceives these to be the dangerous tendencies implicit in our cultural assumptions about the meaning of life and death. In contrast, I am less concerned about these matters that, so long as meaningful discussions continue, will be subject to a constant process of rethinking and correction. Instead what worries me more are conceptual approaches that, however appealing, threaten to erode our ability to reason and discuss these matters clearly. I would urge Leon Kass to rethink his presuppositions and methodology, without in the process losing the keen sensitivity that animates his moral concern.

NOTES AND REFERENCES

1.   For a powerful discussion of the operation of these coercive forces in a real social setting, see Richard Fenigsen, "A Case Against Dutch Euthanasia," *Hastings Center Report* 19, 1 (January/February 1989): 22–30.

2.   See especially his *The Nazi Doctors* (New York: Basic Books, 1986) for an intensive development of the way in which medically authorized "mercy killing" led to programs of mass extermination.

3.   Some have argued that we must distinguish between the Nazi experience of medically authorized killing and what might transpire in a society where euthanasia is regulated by law. See, for example, Daniel Callahan, "Can We Return To Disease?" *Hastings Center Report* 19, 1 (January/February 1989): 5. This experiment, however, seems to me too perilous to duplicate.

4.   Garrett Hardin, "The Tragedy of the Commons," *Science* 162 (1968): 1233–1248.

5.   Former Colorado Governor Richard Lamm has had his name associated with this unfortunate idea. *New York Times,* March 29, 1984, p. A16.

9

Ethics and the Epidemic of HIV Infection

LeRoy Walters

A TALE OF TWO RESEARCH PROTOCOLS ON HIV INFECTION, AIDS-RELATED COMPLEX (ARC), AND AIDS

In August of 1987, the National Institutes of Health initiated two large clinical trials to compare the effectiveness of one drug, azidothymidine (AZT), with placebo pills. One study, called 016, sought to recruit patients with one or two early symptoms of the so-called "AIDS-related complex," or ARC. These symptoms might be weight loss, a chronic rash, or persistent diarrhea. The other study, called 019, enrolled people who are clearly infected with the human immunodeficiency virus (HIV) but who have not yet experienced any major symptoms of their infection.

I have had the privilege of sitting on the Data and Safety Monitoring Board for these two studies, as well as for several other studies, since 1986. The major role of such a board is to review the interim results of such studies, so that the studies can be stopped or modified as soon as a meaningful conclusion has been reached. In the first part of my essay, I will discuss some of the ethical issues faced by the board as it tried to decide, in August of this year [1989], whether to recommend the termination of these two large randomized clinical trials.

Protocol 016

At its August 1–2 meeting the board had information on study 016 through July 21. A total of 713 patients had been enrolled in this study during the preceding 23 months. The average length of time that these patients had been in the study was 9 months. Of these 713 patients, 515 already had somewhat compromised functioning in their immune systems. That is, when they entered the study, they had CD4 (or T4) counts between 200 and 500.

The data presented to the board on August 1 and 2 showed that 50 of the 713 patients in Protocol 016 had experienced an initial "critical event" during the time of their participation in the study—that is, they had either died or developed full-blown AIDS or progressed to more advanced AIDS-related complex. Here is how the critical events were distributed between the group treated with AZT and the group treated with placebo.

Treatment E	Treatment F
36 events	14 events

Source: Division of AIDS, National Institute of Allergy and Infectious Diseases, National Institutes of Health, and the AIDS Clinical Trials Group.

Another way of looking at the study results to date was to ask: What were the probabilities that any given high-risk patient in this trial would enjoy 15 months of failure-free survival—that is, would live and would not experience progression of his or her disease? Here again the comparative figures strongly favored Treatment F.

But what about toxic side effects of treatment with AZT? The board was pleased to note that less than 5% of patients assigned to either treatment experienced major toxicity. That figure is much lower than the 30–40% of patients with full-blown AIDS who experience serious side effects with AZT.

In short, all of the comparisons the board saw showed a clear advantage for Treatment F over Treatment E, and neither treatment produced toxic side effects in large numbers of patients. Thus, even though the study was less than half finished, according to the original timetable, the difference between the two treatments was so great that it was still statistically significant. The board members then asked themselves: Is Treatment F the active drug or the placebo? At that point we "unblinded" ourselves, determined that Treatment F was indeed AZT, and voted to recommend stopping the trial on ethical grounds. In our view, the superiority of AZT to placebo was sufficiently clear that it would be ethically inappropriate to continue administering placebo tablets to patients in this study.

On August 3, one day after the board made its recommendation, the Department of Health and Human Services issued a press release summarizing the results of the study. The following day, August 4, both the *New York Times* and the *Washington Post* carried the news about Protocol 016 in front-page stories.

Protocol 019

The board was simultaneously overseeing a second study, this one involving people who already had been infected with the human immunodeficiency virus but who had as yet experienced no serious symptoms. Protocol 019, as this study was called, involved large numbers of asymptomatic people (who probably should not be called "patients" precisely because they *are* without symptoms). By July of this year 3,200 people had been recruited to this study in 32 treatment units. Study participants were randomly assigned to one of three groups: a placebo group, a group receiving a low dose of AZT (500 mg per day), and a group receiving a high dose of AZT (1,500 mg per day). The study was designed to show whether AZT helped to prevent or at least delay the progression of HIV infection into more serious clinical disease, and, if so, which dose of the drug was on balance better. The average follow-up time for people in this study was more than 1 year when the data were analyzed.

At its early August meeting, the Data Safety and Monitoring Board had information on 2,808 persons who had been asymptomatic at the time they had entered the study. Fewer than 100 of these people had experienced progression of their HIV infection—to AIDS, to advanced "AIDS-related complex," or to death. Most of the people whose condition had worsened had CD4 counts of 500 or less when they had entered the study. The designers of the study had planned for separate analyses of this higher risk subgroup, and because such a large proportion of the progressions had indeed occurred in this subgroup, the board paid particular attention to the fate of these people.

In this case, the board members were unblinded immediately; that is, we were told by the statisticians which patients who had progressed had received placebo tablets, which had received the low dose of AZT, and which had received the high dose of AZT. In the higher risk group, the people who had entered the study with CD4 counts less than 500, we thought we saw a clear pattern favoring AZT, especially the *lower* dose of AZT over placebo. (See Table 1 for precise figures on disease progression in the three treatment groups.)

There was just one small fly in the ointment. It was early August, and the data that the board was examining had been "frozen" as of May 10, almost 3 months earlier. Further, the average interval between the last contact with subjects and the freezing of the data base had been 34 days. Thus, the study results that the board was examining were almost 4 months old. Board members were concerned that a few additional events in the interim, especially if they were clustered in one of the two groups receiving AZT, might radically change the picture presented in Table 1.

Table 1.   HIV Progression by Treatment Group:
CD4 < 500 Stratum

Treatment Group	Number of Patients	Number of Progressions	Progression Rate [a]
Placebo	428	31	7.5
500 mg	453	8	2.1
1500 mg	457	12	3.4

[a] Failures per 100 person-years of observation.
Source: Division of AIDS, National Institute of Allergy and Infectious Diseases, National Institutes of Health, and the AIDS Clinical Trials Group.

Thus, despite the board's interest in terminating Study 019 as soon as a definitive result was reached, we asked the statistical coordinating centers tracking this study to gather as much additional information as possible about events that might have occurred between early April and early August of 1989. The statistical centers and the board agreed that the updated figures would be sent to the board by Federal Express or Express Mail within a few weeks of the meeting, that board members would each review the new data, and that a conference call would then be held to reach a final decision on possibly recommending termination of this important study. The statistical coordinating centers must have worked night and day during the next 2 weeks. On August 14, less than 2 weeks after the conclusion of the previous board meeting, a 15-page updated analysis was sent to the board. At 11 A.M. on August 16 the board "met" by conference call. One board member was on a camping trip in Colorado. Our chairman was poised to leave on a trip to Sweden. Our Pacific Coast member had to rise very early to prepare for his participation in the deliberations. I was on vacation by a quiet lake in western Pennsylvania. But we were all on-line for more than an hour of intensive discussion on that August morning.

The key table in the updated analysis was the one that corresponded to the earlier Table 1. In the interim since August 2, the principal investigator for the study and the statistical coordinating centers had discovered 23 new events in the high-risk subgroup with CD4 counts less than 500. These events could now be added to the events reported earlier and would give the board a much firmer basis for its judgment. The critical information appears in Table 2 (an update of Table 1).

Table 2. HIV Progression by Treatment Group:
CD4 < 500 Stratum (Updated)

Treatment Group	Number of Patients	Number of Progressions	Progression Rate [a]
Placebo	428	38	7.6
500 mg	453	17	3.6
1500 mg	457	19	4.2

[a] Failures per 100 person-years of observation.
Source: Division of AIDS, National Institute of Allergy and Infectious Diseases, National Institutes of Health, and the AIDS Clinical Trials Group.

What these updated numbers showed is that AZT in both dosages continued to have an advantage over placebo. The difference between the 500-mg dose of AZT and placebo was statistically significant, even if one adjusts for the early stage of the study. (The actual comparison, based on a logrank test, was $p = .003$.)

The board also examined life-table plots that reflect the interval of time until treatment failure occurred in the high-risk group. I am not at liberty to discuss the details of these life-table plots until the scientific paper on Protocol 019 is published by the researchers who conducted the study. What I can say is that a delay in the progression of an infection can be either temporary or permanent. For some participants in Protocol 019, the drug AZT provided only temporary protection from the destructive power of the human immunodeficiency virus.

Again in this study the board looked at the question of toxic side effects. Among the high-risk subjects who received the higher dose of AZT, about 12% developed some kind of serious side effects in hemoglobin levels or blood cells. For the comparable low-dose AZT group this figure was only about 3% and for the placebo group about 2%. Nausea was reported by 3–5% of high-risk study participants taking AZT, regardless of dose level, and by virtually no one who had been randomly assigned to placebo.

On the basis of this updated analysis, the Data and Safety Monitoring Board voted unanimously to recommend terminating the administration of placebo to patients in the high-risk (<500 CD4) group. The recommendation of the board was reported by Secretary of Health and Human Services Louis Sullivan at a news briefing the next day, August 17, and was a front-page story in the *New York Times* and the *Washington Post* on the following day.

THE PUBLIC INTERPRETATION OF THE DATA
FROM THE TWO PROTOCOLS

In the press release that announced the termination of the first study, Protocol 019, Secretary Sullivan was quoted as follows: "We are on the threshold of a time when advances in biomedical research will enable HIV-infected individuals to live longer, more comfortable lives." Dr. Anthony Fauci, Director of the National Institute of Allergy and Infectious Diseases, was quoted as saying: "For the first time, the benefits of antiretroviral treatment for patients with early symptomatic HIV infection have been clearly shown. In this study, significantly fewer persons receiving zidovudine [AZT] progressed to advanced ARC or AIDS. This finding could extend treatment to an estimated one to two thousand persons with early symptoms of HIV infection. It also emphasizes how critical it is that persons at risk for HIV infection be tested and seek prompt medical care." The headline writers at the *New York Times* translated these statements as follows: "Strong Evidence That AZT Holds Off AIDS." The *Washington Post* announced: "Early AIDS Treatment Urged: AZT Found Helpful When Symptoms Begin."

On August 17 at the briefing that announced the termination of Protocol 019 for high-risk people, a press release was distributed. In the press release Secretary Sullivan was quoted as saying: "Today we are witnessing an additional milestone in the battle to change AIDS from a fatal disease to a treatable one." Dr. Sullivan continued, "These results provide real hope for the millions of people worldwide who are infected with HIV." Dr. Fauci was a bit more cautious. In the press release he was quoted as follows: "This study has clearly demonstrated that early treatment with zidovudine [AZT] can slow disease progression without significant side effects in HIV-infected persons with fewer than 500 T4 cells who do not yet have symptoms." The next day the *New York Times* carried the following headline at the upper left on the front page: "Drug Said to Help AIDS Cases with Virus but No Symptoms." According to the headline on the front page of the *Washington Post*, "AZT Found to Delay Onset of AIDS; Treatment Urged for Up to 650,000."

Researchers and activists quoted in the four newspaper stories warmly welcomed the news of success in the two studies. For example, Richard Dunne, executive director of the Gay Men's Health Crisis Center in New York, commented that the results from Protocol 016 put AIDS treatment into "a new age." He added, however, that the next challenge would be to "develop plans and resources in a very short period of time to deliver this information and follow it up with services." Members of the U.S. Congress were also pleased but voiced concern about the problem of access to the drug AZT. Henry Waxman, Chairman of the House Energy and Commerce subcommittee on health, commented to the *Washington Post:* "It's wonderful news that there is something to keep infected people from getting sick. . . . But it's not enough to develop a drug; we must also get it to people who need it."[1] According to the *Post*, Waxman called for the manufacturer of AZT, Burroughs Wellcome Company, to lower the price of AZT, which averages $8,000 per year for each of the approximately 30,000 patients who currently take it in the United States. The *Post* story continued: "David Barry, the company's vice president for science, said Burroughs Wellcome will keep evaluating prices, 'noting the potential for increased patient numbers.' "[2]

Here I would simply inject a note of caution. Everyone who cares about people with HIV infection and about controlling the current epidemic has been waiting for some good news for a long time. There is at least a danger that the positive results of Protocols 016 and 019 will be overinterpreted. We have already seen that some people on AZT in both studies nonetheless experienced progression of their infection. I have also suggested that in Protocol 019 the benefit provided by AZT may have been temporary; that is, the drug delayed but did not ultimately prevent progression to more serious symptoms. Thus, we have only taken the first few steps in a journey that may turn out to be a hundred miles long.

IMPLICATIONS OF THE STUDY RESULTS

For Research

These two studies, Protocols 016 and 019, once again demonstrate the potential value of placebo-controlled randomized clinical trials in a situation where there is genuine uncertainty about the effectiveness and toxicity of a new treatment. The review process and the early termination of at least part of each study reflects the importance of periodic monitoring of such studies by an impartial and independent board.

As noted earlier, the clinical success of AZT in these two studies was real but limited. Not all study participants who took AZT were helped by the drug, and there may be a time limitation on the capacity of AZT to ward off the progression of disease. Thus, if anything, the promising results of these studies point to the need for redoubled efforts in research. Scientists need to develop and test even better treatments; if possible, they should develop a safe and effective vaccine, like the vaccine that is now available for hepatitis B. These research efforts will require a strong national commitment and, no less importantly, substantial funding.

Another important implication of the study results, in my view, is that no new placebo-controlled studies should be planned at this time for HIV-infected people with CD4 counts less than 500. Rather, new studies should compare the safety and effectiveness of AZT with another potentially helpful drug. If the new drug turns out to be safer and more efficacious than AZT, that new drug should then be the standard of comparison in the next study, and so on.

However, two other related questions about research remain somewhat perplexing to me. The first is: What should happen to similar randomized clinical trials that are currently ongoing? For example, the Veterans Administration is conducting a placebo-controlled trial that is quite similar in design to Protocol 016, although in a somewhat different patient population. Should that trial be continued or stopped? Would our answer depend in part on whether the study results converge with or diverge from the results in Protocol 016? My second perplexing question is in some ways the obverse side of the first: In how many different studies should a particular conclusion be reached before we accept it as definitive? Is one well-designed study sufficient, or should we require two or even more studies that concur in their results?

For Public Health

As we noted earlier, Dr. Fauci saw a clear public-health implication in the results of Protocol 016. In his view, the study findings "[emphasize] how critical it is that persons at risk for HIV infection be tested and seek prompt medical care." Dr. Fauci reiterated this point at the press briefing on Protocol 019 in mid-August. What ethical arguments can be advanced in support of Dr. Fauci's recommendation, and are there ethical counterarguments?

To give this recommendation the careful scrutiny it deserves, we would need to clarify first who the "persons at risk for HIV infection" are and thus how many people would need to be tested if the recommendation were universally followed. Presumably intravenous drug users who share needles would be near the top of the list, as would people who have engaged in unprotected receptive anal intercourse with multiple sexual partners. It is less clear whether every recipient of a blood transfusion since 1977 or every person who has had any kind of sexual intercourse with more than one partner since 1977 should also be considered "at risk."

Let us assume for the moment that we can identify a group of people who are "at risk," or perhaps "at substantial risk," for HIV infection. How does the decision about whether to be tested look to the individual at risk, in light of the results from Protocols 016 and 019? If we try to stand in the shoes of that person, we find ourselves balancing potential medical benefits against potential social harms. The monologue might go somewhat as follows:

> If I am tested and test positive, my physician (assuming I have one) can monitor my health status and prescribe AZT if my number of T4 cells dips below 500. Also, if I get a lung infection, the physician can offer me aerosolized pentamidine, which seems quite effective. And I should hear immediately of any new treatments that are developed.
>
> On the other hand, if I am tested, I will have to report the fact of having been tested the next time I am asked the question—even if my test discovers no infection. In the eyes of some people and organizations, agreeing to be tested is already an admission of guilt. If my test is positive, how can I be sure that that information will be kept confidential? Can I be confident that my results will not be leaked to my employer, my landlord, or insurance companies—with potentially serious consequences? Even worse, how can I be assured that my spouse (or intimate friends) will not find out?

I conclude that for an at-risk individual, *either* a decision to be tested *or* a decision not to be tested can be a rational decision, given the current social context.

In the preceding soliloquy, the hypothetical speaker focused on self-regarding reasons for and against being tested. Ethics, however, deals with our obligations to others as well as with our own rights and interests. The major other-regarding reason for being tested is that, if one discovers that one is infected, one can take measures that reduce the probability of infecting others. However, as of last year there were no published studies demonstrating that knowledge of antibody status, whether positive or negative, in fact caused heterosexual men or women to practice safer sex.[3]

Until this point, we have been thinking about HIV-antibody testing on a personal level. This question can and should also be analyzed at the level of public policy. What implications, if any, do the results from Protocols 016 and 019 have for ethically acceptable public policymaking?

First, now that a drug has been developed that is potentially useful to large numbers of HIV-infected but asymptomatic people, existing social barriers to testing should be removed. Specifically, clear public policies should be developed and enforced that guarantee the confidentiality of testing and test results and that prohibit discrimination against tested or antibody-positive people. Several of the states have led the way in this regard, and the Justice Department of the federal government has done a constructive about-face in its position on discrimination against HIV-infected people. But much more work remains to be done.

Second, programs of voluntary testing should be attractive to larger numbers of people because they can now see a tangible benefit from early detection of infection and careful monitoring of CD4 counts. As even better treatments are developed, there will be even less need—and even less justification—for mandatory testing programs among adults. (Infants are a special case here. As improved testing methods and better therapies are developed, it is possible that mandatory infant screening programs will become morally justifiable, at least in areas with a high prevalence of infection. The model for such programs would be existing programs that screen newborn infants for genetic diseases like phenylketonuria and hypothyroidism.[4])

Third, it is not immediately clear what priority ought to be assigned to testing programs in the allocation of public funds. We have already considered the critical need for additional high-quality research on HIV infection and its prevention and treatment. Within the public-health arena, should more money now be allocated to testing, or are skillfully prepared and explicit programs of general public education more important? Alternatively, would it be more cost-effective to invest available funds in treatment programs for intravenous drug users, providing treatment on demand, as the Presidential Commission on the HIV Epidemic strongly recommended?[5] (That Commission recommended the development of 2,500 new treatment facilities for drug users and the addition of almost 60,000 new workers in these facilities.)

The Delivery of Health Care

The development of new drugs like AZT will, in the short run, exacerbate fundamental problems in the United States health care delivery "system." Even before the current epidemic 15 to 17.5% of United States residents under age 65 lacked both public and private health insurance. These percentages translate into 30 to 35 million Americans. An additional 10 to 15% of those under 65 who are insured are not adequately protected against serious or long-term illness.[6] The thought of complicating this situation with major new expenditures for perhaps half a million people at perhaps $5,000 per year for medication alone staggers the imagination. (My home calculator could not handle these figures. The added cost would come to $2.5 billion per year.)

The epidemic of HIV infection and AIDS is increasingly concentrated on people of color and people who either were poor or who became poor as a result of becoming ill. Forty percent of all people with full-blown AIDS receive at least partial coverage for the costs of their illness from

Medicaid, a federal–state program for poor people. In locations like New York and New Jersey, the proportion of Medicaid recipients may be as high as 65 to 70%. For hospitals providing care to people with AIDS, Medicaid is now the principal source of payment.[7] As a society, we have not yet really confronted the central moral question: Do we believe that every individual has a moral right to an adequate level of health care? If we do, then we will be dissatisfied with the current patchwork, or, to change the metaphor, with a safety net that includes so many gaping holes.

The choice is, in a way, quite simple. We can either respond to the people who are infected with HIV or we can write them off as not deserving of our care. If we reform our approach to health care to include this large cohort of our fellow citizens, we may find that we are also more creative and effective in meeting the needs of many other groups of poor, disabled, and chronically ill human beings. And if we tackle the problem of equitable access to health care, perhaps we would move on to confront some of the root causes of our current distress— especially poverty and urban decay.

Admiral James Watkins, now the Secretary of the U.S. Department of Energy, chaired the Presidential Commission on the HIV Epidemic. Admiral Watkins went into the commission's study process attempting to understand how to cope with a public health problem. He came out of the process with a vision of new possibilities for our society. In the transmittal letter that accompanied the commission's report, Admiral Watkins wrote:

> While we found it a grave tragedy, we also saw the HIV epidemic as an opportunity to confront and begin to solve many of the problems our society faces. We saw an opportunity to begin to eliminate flaws in our health care system resulting in a better life for all Americans; we saw an opportunity to begin to educate our young people about their own human biology so that they can better appreciate the unique worth and dignity of themselves and others; we saw an opportunity to begin to eliminate discrimination against persons with HIV infection, as well as persons with other disabilities and illnesses, and embrace them as part of the mainstream of American life; we saw an opportunity to begin to turn the goodness that is out there, just waiting to be harnessed into an unbeatable army against this viral enemy that has captured early ground.[8]

NOTES AND REFERENCES

1. *The Washington Post*, August 4, 1989, A18.
2. *Ibid.*

3.   Institute of Medicine, National Academy of Sciences, *Confronting AIDS: Update 1988* (Washington, D.C.: National Academy Press, 1988), 75.

4.   Lori B. Andrews, comp., *State Laws and Regulations Governing Newborn Screening* (Chicago: American Bar Association, 1985).

5.   Presidential Commission on the Human Immunodeficiency Virus Epidemic, *Report* (Washington, D.C.: U.S. Government Printing Office, June 1988), 94–98, 171.

6.   LeRoy Walters, "Ethical Issues in the Prevention and Treatment of HIV Infection and AIDS," *Science* 239 (February 5, 1988): 597–603.

7.   Institute of Medicine, *op. cit.*, 111.

8.   Presidential Commission, *op. cit.*, vi.

10

Obstacles and Opportunities in Responding to the Epidemic of HIV Infection: A Response to LeRoy Walters

Carol Levine

With his customary clarity, precision, and sensitivity, LeRoy Walters has described the ethical deliberations of the Data Safety and Monitoring Board (DSMB) that reviewed the data on two AZT protocols, 016 (which enrolled patients with early symptoms of HIV infection) and 019 (which enrolled HIV-infected asymptomatic patients). As a member of a similar board created by another branch of the National Institute of Allergy and Infectious Diseases (NIAID), I am particularly grateful for his "insider's view" of the DSMB's decision-making process.

His presentation reminds us that bioethics plays an important role in research and policy decisions as well as clinical ones, and that not all mortal choices concern a single individual or a family's fate. In this case the DSMB's decisions will affect all people infected with HIV—an estimated million Americans.

Since I agree in large measure with Dr. Walters' conclusions, in my commentary I would like to take one step backward and one step forward. The step backward will describe the context for the regulation of human subjects research that prevails in the United States today; the step forward will amplify Dr. Walter's comments on the research, medical practice, and policy implications of releasing these data at this time.

RESEARCH AS A BENEFIT, NOT JUST A RISK

There is an extraordinary pressure to develop effective therapies against AIDS. This pressure, along with other societal and political movements that have set in motion waves of deregulation, will affect the way all drugs are developed, tested, and marketed.

Only a decade ago critics of the therapeutic drug approval process complained about a "drug lag." Because of the strict regulations of the Food and Drug Administration (FDA), many drugs came to market abroad long before they were approved for American patients. Today the pendulum has swung so far that many people are worried about a "drug leap." Driven by the urgency of finding treatments for people with AIDS and HIV disease, the FDA has let down the regulatory barriers. In a process called "parallel track," promising but largely untested drugs will be made available to desperate patients who are ineligible for or do not have access to controlled clinical trials.

The current system of regulation of human subjects research and the drug approval process was a reaction to scandal and abuse. Modern concern with the ethics of human subjects research began with the revelations at the Doctors' Trial in Nuremberg of the most horrific abuse under the Nazis of human rights and dignity. One of the pioneers of concern for the ethics of human subjects research in this country, psychiatrist Jay Katz, wrote a few years ago in explaining his early interest in this subject: "I had lost most of my cousins, aunts, and uncles in the Holocaust. How many of them, I wondered, had been condemned to participation in these experiments?"[1] A year or so ago I reread some of the transcripts of that trial. It is a sobering experience, especially when one remembers that the perpetrators of these atrocities were not SS guards but some of the most respected members of the German medical and scientific worlds. A recent study by Dr. Robert Berger has demonstrated that the infamous hypothermia experiments at Dachau were not only inhumane but also scientifically worthless.[2]

The Nazi revelations were followed by other scandals, none so egregious but still profoundly disturbing. In the early 1960s in Europe and Australia thousands of pregnant women were given thalidomide as a sedative; many of their babies were born horribly deformed. That disaster was largely avoided in the United States by a cautious FDA official's refusal to accept the drug companies' safety data. In 1966 Henry Knowles Beecher, a highly respected Harvard anesthesiologist, published an eye-opening article describing many examples of research studies in the United States that involved high levels of risk and low levels of voluntariness and consent.[3]

The resulting wave of justifiable professional and public concern led to restrictive regulations. Research involving prisoners has all but ended. Women and members of minority groups are underrepresented in drug trials, even for conditions that affect them. Pediatricians have to prescribe many drugs for infants and young children on the basis of adult data because, as drug labels typically warn, "few studies have been carried out in this group."

AIDS is contributing to a reexamination of these policies. But while the headlines focus on speeding up the drug approval process, another, quieter revolution is underway. Many people who were previously considered too vulnerable to be research subjects are precisely the ones who stand most to benefit from being in trials. Pregnant women and women of childbearing age, infants and children, prisoners, current or former drug users, members of racial or ethnic minority groups, poor people—all these are groups traditionally excluded from research trials but all hard hit by AIDS and HIV.

But the landscape is changing. For example, the ban on research involving prisoners has been partially lifted. The federal regulations never excluded the possibility of including prisoners in trials for medical conditions that they themselves suffered from, but in practice prison authorities avoided any research involving inmates. California has had the most restrictive law on the books, which declares categorically: "No biomedical research shall be conducted on any prisoner in this state." On September 29, 1989, Governor Dukmejian enacted a bill that found that "state law designed to protect prisoners from inappropriate medical experimentation has had the unintended effect of preventing prisoners from having access to drugs or treatments which might be required for good medical care." The new law will "provide prisoners access to certain investigational drugs or treatments on the same basis that they are made available to patients outside the prison setting."[4]

The *Los Angeles Times* reported in September 1989 that blacks and Latinos, who make up 42% of the adult AIDS patients in the United States account for only 20.4% of subjects enrolled in the trials run by the National Institute of Allergy and Infectious Diseases (NIAID). Only 11.3% of the participants in the federal studies are intravenous drug users; yet they account for 27.5% of adult AIDS patients, and the percentage is growing.[5]

The information about dosage and side effects obtained in drug trials in middle-class gay white men may not be applicable to women, children, and poor minority drug users. It is scientifically as well as ethically important to include all affected groups in trials.

There are obvious hurdles. Many potential subjects lack access to primary care, the traditional route of referral to research, and to health insurance to pay for costs of care other than the drug itself, which is free to trial participants. Many subjects do not live near the academic centers where most research is conducted; they may need money for transportation and child care in order to participate. Many may be suspicious of research, particularly when access to primary health care is inadequate.

"Why do researchers come to us only when they want to try out something new?" one potential subject asked. "Why don't they give us
standard care first?"

These barriers are being overcome through extensive outreach efforts
and greater sensitivity. In New York City, for example, three major medical centers have 40% or more minority participation in AIDS trials, and
community-based research is becoming a much more accessible alternative to academic center trials.

Institutional Review Boards (IRBs)—the committees that review research protocols for compliance with ethical standards—are also looking
more closely at exclusion and inclusion criteria. The IRB of New York
City's Community Research Initiative, for instance, requests investigators to use a standard of "ability to comply with the protocol" rather
than automatically excluding drug users because they are assumed to be
unreliable.

Women of childbearing age with AIDS or HIV infection suffer from
triple jeopardy. They are excluded because many of them fit into three
categories researchers and drug companies want to avoid: potentially
pregnant females, members of minority groups, and intravenous drug
users.

IRBs are beginning to look more closely at the justification for excluding women—whether it is simply automatic risk avoidance or whether
there is a scientific rationale for believing that the particular trial poses
clear and unacceptable risks to the woman or a potential or actual fetus
that outweigh the benefits.

Some trials involving children have already been conducted, and the
federal Department of Health and Human Service's Work Group on
Pediatric HIV Infection and Disease has strongly endorsed expanded
research on children. It said: "Because pediatric HIV disease differs from
adult disease, it is necessary to conduct innovative experimental research designed specifically for children. . . . Medical tradition and current FDA guidelines, which restrict testing of new agents and protocols
in children until at least some safety data have been collected for adults,
will have to be reconsidered. . . ."[6]

In New Jersey, which is second only to New York in the number of
pediatric AIDS cases in the nation, a statewide Pediatric AIDS Advisory
Committee has urged states to reevaluate their current policies and procedures "to ensure that HIV-infected children who are wards of the
State can participate in appropriate clinical trials and treatment, with all
the protection accorded to any child."[7]

Although trials involving sick children, whatever their disease, are
among the most troubling for IRBs to review, trials involving asymptomatic HIV-infected infants present additional ethical challenges. Given the
current state of technology, it is impossible to tell which babies who test

positive for HIV from birth until the age of about 15 months are truly infected. A positive HIV antibody test in a newborn is evidence of HIV infection in the mother; given current experience, about a third of the babies with antibodies are themselves infected, and two-thirds will lose the antibodies in the first year or so of life. This means of course that in a trial of a toxic substance with unknown long-term effects on development or health, two-thirds of the subjects will not even have the condition the drug is intended to treat. Some IRBs have already approved such protocols; others may find the risks to the healthy subjects outweigh the potential benefits to the infected babies.

Expanding subject selection to include the people who will be taking the drugs once they are approved makes good sense, not just in AIDS, but in other diseases as well. However, the current standards of consent, confidentiality, and voluntariness as well as the special protections for vulnerable subjects such as prisoners and children must be maintained. It is in fact the existence of protections that has made research less risky and more respectful of subjects' rights.

Before I turn to other implications of the AZT data described by Dr. Walters, let me respond briefly to the two questions about further research on AZT that he raises in his paper. He asks: "What should happen to similar randomized clinical trials that are currently ongoing?" In Europe similar trials of AZT on asymptomatic patients have not been stopped on the basis of the American findings. I suggest that the Data Safety and Monitoring Board of the ongoing trial review its data to date. If it shows a similar, substantial benefit for those on AZT, the trial should be stopped. If it does not, it should be continued. However, the subjects should be informed that there is preliminary evidence from another trial that AZT does confer benefit on some (but not all) patients; this seems to me to be relevant information to their decision to continue to participate.

On the second question, "In how many different studies should a particular conclusion be reached before we accept it as definitive?" there is no single answer. Since both protocols 016 and 019 enrolled large numbers of subjects, the evidence is quite convincing. However, since they were mainly gay white men, the results may not be applicable to other populations, and a second study may give even more precise results. As Dr. Walters suggests, it would not be ethically justifiable to start new placebo-controlled trials to examine the same question, but it would be ethically justifiable to continue ongoing ones if subjects agree.

EARLY INTERVENTION

Let me turn now to the policy implications of the announcement of the unblinding of the 016 and 019 AZT protocols. "Early intervention" has become the slogan of doctors, patients, patient advocates, and public health officers. Yet, as Dr. Walters pointed out, the overwhelmingly positive press response to the announcements may have overstated the optimistic view. It is precisely when medicine's capacity to enhance patient welfare appears to be increasing that there is a danger that important ethical concerns can be overridden or disregarded.

Early identification and intervention offer clear benefits. Dr. Walters has stated some of them. Beyond starting AZT treatment when the immune system starts to falter, there is the possibility of preventing or delaying the onset of *Pneumocystis carinii* pneumonia, the most common infection and the one most often associated with early death, by the use of aerosolized pentamidine. Another benefit is the opportunity to test for other diseases—tuberculosis and syphilis, for example—and to institute appropriate prophylaxis or therapies. Many people who learn that they are HIV positive are motivated to engage in healthier lifestyles—changing their diets, exercising more, and reducing cigarette, alcohol, and drug use.

However, there are medical risks in the early administration of a toxic drug to which some patients are already developing resistance. No one knows the long-term effects—it seems that there is a finite period of AZT efficacy. Does early intervention reduce the likelihood of efficacy when symptoms do develop?

Dr. Walters mentioned some of the social risks of being identified as HIV positive. In addition to the possibility of discrimination, early intervention is an expensive proposition. Most of the costs of drugs and outpatient care are not covered by insurance, and even if they are, patients are often unwilling to file claims out of fear that they will lose coverage for the even more costly hospital stays that may occur in the future.

One of the risks of being identified as HIV positive is that it may be difficult to obtain health care. Few community physicians are willing to care for HIV-infected patients, out of fear of transmission or fear that the rest of their practice will suffer if it becomes known that they treat HIV-infected patients or out of a belief that they should not have to treat patients who have engaged in risky behaviors of which they disapprove. Despite the consistent views against such discrimination expressed by all the major medical organizations, the reality is that many physicians do not want to care for HIV-infected patients, and that the ones who do are overburdened already.

In sum, the benefit–risk calculus has many elements. Treatment for asymptomatic HIV infection is still evolving, costly, and with significant long-term risks. But AIDS is still ultimately a fatal disease, and early intervention offers both the potential of prolonging life and the psychological benefit of giving individuals a sense of control over their destinies. Given such uncertainty, patients, in consultation with their physicians, will weigh the various elements differently. Some will choose an aggressive, all-out approach; others will select certain treatments and not others; and some may prefer to watch and wait.

For individuals to have the opportunity to make the best personal, voluntary, and informed choice, there are now clinical and ethical grounds for establishing voluntary anonymous or confidential screening programs in settings where individuals who may have been infected with HIV are treated. If that is so, why not make HIV testing mandatory or at least "routine"—that is, administered without any specific discussion or consent? In fact, some public health officials and others are advocating just such policies. Whereas mandatory screening failed to gain wide acceptance among public health officials on the grounds of the harm principle—preventing transmission to others—it may well succeed on the grounds of beneficence—promoting patient welfare. The target populations have changed. In the early years of the epidemic, mandatory screening proposals were aimed at gay men; now they are aimed at pregnant women and newborns. There is no justification for mandatory screening of adults on the grounds of therapeutic benefit. Mandatory, that is, legally required or institutionally enforced, screening for early intervention for competent adults would be a major departure from the accepted standards of medical practice. In our legal and ethical systems, competent adults have the ultimate decision-making authority over their medical care. Despite the well-documented clinical benefits of screening for other potentially fatal diseases—breast cancer, for example—screening programs are entirely voluntary. Changing this standard because of the infectious and stigmatized nature of HIV disease would be a grave mistake.

If there were an intervention that both benefited an infected person and also prevented transmission by rendering him or her noninfectious, mandatory screening might be considered and might be justified on the basis of the harm principle. But even in that entirely hypothetical situation, the likelihood of public health benefit would have to be weighed against the possible side effects and the intrusive and long-term nature of the intervention. Since HIV is transmitted through behavior that can be modified, clinical intervention is not the only possible means of controlling the spread of infection.

The case of newborns presents a more complex situation. Infants cannot consent for themselves, and society has an obligation to ensure that they are not deprived of potentially life-saving therapeutic benefits. Nevertheless, the welfare of children is assumed in general to be most effectively protected by deferring to parents. Although respect for persons is usually considered to be a principle affecting individuals, family autonomy has a long legal and moral tradition as well.

Unlike the situation with competent adults, there are mandatory or quasimandatory newborn screening programs in place for a few conditions. Screening for phenylketonuria (PKU), for example, is mandated in most states. In the case of PKU, there is a definitive test to identify the rare infant with the genetic enzyme deficiency that prevents the metabolization of phenylalanine. There is a well-established therapeutic regimen—a diet low in phenylalanine—that is highly effective in preventing retardation. It must be initiated early in infancy and continued until the child is 5 or older.

Unlike the cases of PKU, however, there is at present no definitive screening test to identify the HIV-infected infant, no proven therapy, and no proven benefits to early intervention. There are also strong arguments *against* mandatory HIV screening at present. Mandatory screening of all newborns would entail the coercive identification of infected mothers, since the HIV antibodies in the infant reveal infection in the mother. These women are typically from minority communities. Often they are poor and have a history of drug use. They are particularly subject to attempts to override their parental rights. Unless specifically demonstrated to be unable to act in their child's best interests, mothers at high risk for HIV infection should have the power to exercise the rights accorded to other parents, including the right to refuse HIV testing for their infants.

Dr. Walters suggests that mandatory screening for newborns may be ethically justifiable. I suggest that will occur only when a definitive test that accurately identifies HIV-infected infants becomes available and when a treatment has been demonstrated to be safe and effective in prolonging life and improving its quality for the child; only then will overriding parental refusal for HIV testing be ethically defensible on the basis of the harm principle.

Screening programs to identify asymptomatic individuals for clinical purposes that do not at the same time plan for appropriate follow-up services fail to meet the ethical standards of justice or beneficence. The demands of justice go beyond a prohibition of discrimination. They require a systematic and full-scale commitment to planning for and providing the medical and social services that will be required to meet the needs of HIV-infected individuals.

With over 150,000 cases of CDC-defined AIDS reported as of September 30, 1990, one-third of them in the New York City–northern New Jersey region, the health care systems in heavily affected areas have been severely strained.[8] Providing experimental and therapeutic regimens as well as careful monitoring for the estimated one million asymptomatic individuals with HIV infection will require a dramatic expansion of services. If the majority of asymptomatic seropositive people were treated on the basis of the current Public Health Service recommendations, costs would run into the billions of dollars.

When HIV antibody testing first became available in mid-1985, its primary function was to prevent the spread of infection through the screening of blood, and, in conjunction with counseling, to foster behavior change. Out of the many sharp debates that surrounded the test at the time, a broad alliance of clinicians, public health officials, political leaders, and AIDS activists forged a consensus that stressed the importance of specific informed consent for testing and the protection of the confidentiality of the test results.

The next phase of the HIV epidemic will thus be marked by improvements in therapies and by profound challenges to the ethical principles that should govern the practice of medicine and public health. Only if careful consideration is given to the rights of individuals, to respect for their privacy, and to society's obligations to provide the needed clinical and social services will it be possible to ensure that the cautious optimism that is now medically justified will be translated into policies that are ethically justified.

NOTES AND REFERENCES

1. Jay Katz, "The Regulation of Human Experimentation in the United States—A Personal Odyssey," *IRB* 9, 1 (January/February 1987): 2.

2. Robert L. Berger, "Nazi Science—The Dachau Hypothermia Experiments," *New England Journal of Medicine* 322, 20 (May 17, 1990): 1435–1440.

3. Henry Knowles Beecher, "Ethics and Clinical Research," *New England Journal of Medicine* 274 (1966): 1354–1360.

4. California State Senate Bill No. 452, introduced by Senator Hart, February 13, 1989, and signed into law September 29, 1990.

5. Robert Steinbrook, "AIDS Trials Shortchange Minorities and Drug Users," *The Los Angeles Times*, September 25, 1989.

6. Department of Health and Human Services, *Final Report: Secretary's Work Group on Pediatric HIV Infection and Disease* (Washington D.C.: November 18, 1988): 16.

7. New Jersey Pediatric AIDS Advisory Committee, New Jersey State Department of Health, *Generations in Jeopardy: Responding to HIV Infection in Children, Women, and Adolescents in New Jersey* (September 1989): 16.

8. Centers for Disease Control, *HIV/AIDS Surveillance* (October 1990): 5.

11

Fairness in the Allocation and Delivery of Health Care: The Case of Organ Transplantation

James F. Childress

I have chosen to concentrate on the subject of organ transplantation in an effort not only to make the topic manageable, but also to illuminate a wide range of questions that cannot be discussed in detail. A case study of heart transplantation provides the starting point.

CASE STUDY OF HEART TRANSPLANTATION: ISSUES OF FAIRNESS

Because of the dismal early results of heart transplants following Dr. Christian Barnard's pioneering transplant in 1967, there was a virtual moratorium on the procedure for several years. A few centers in the United States, most notably one at Stanford University, continued heart transplant programs; and by the early 1980s Dr. Norman Shumway and his colleagues at Stanford had achieved good success rates—65% of their carefully selected heart transplant recipients could be expected to survive at least 1 year, and they had a better than 50% chance of surviving 5 years. Because of these results, proponents of cardiac transplantation argued that it should be made widely available, but critics were not convinced that the problem of tissue rejection had been sufficiently solved or that the benefits of cardiac transplantation outweighed its costs.

On February 1, 1980, the 12 lay trustees of the Massachusetts General Hospital announced their decision not to permit heart transplants at that institution "at the present time." Their explanatory statement noted that "to turn away even one potential cardiac transplantation patient is a very trying course to follow," but that "in an age where technology so pervades the medical community, there is a clear responsibility to evaluate new procedures in terms of the greatest good for the greatest number." In June 1980, Patricia Harris, then Secretary of the Department of Health and Human Services (DHHS), withdrew an earlier tentative authorization for Medicare to cover heart transplants, holding that such a technology must be evaluated in terms of its "social consequences" as well as its safety, effectiveness, and acceptance by the medical community. Cost is one social consequence, and the specter of another expensive program like the one for end-stage renal disease, which covers both renal dialysis and transplantation, engendered bureaucratic and congressional caution. For example, the cost of heart transplants at Stanford then averaged more than $100,000 per patient. If 2,000 transplants were performed, the cost would be more than $200 million. If 30,000 transplants were performed, the cost would thus be 3 billion. Estimates vary, but some reports suggest that each year in the United States there may be as many as 35,000 victims of heart disease whose condition is hopeless without cardiac transplantation and who could possibly benefit from cardiac transplantation (if we assume that it would be possible to locate enough hearts for transplantation).

DHHS was also concerned about Stanford's screening criteria, which included "a stable, rewarding family and/or vocational environment to return to post-transplant; a spouse, family member or companion able and willing to make the long-term commitment to provide emotional support before and after the transplant; financial resources to support travel to and from the transplant center accompanied by the family member for final evaluation." "Contraindications" for admission to the waiting list at Stanford included "a history of alcoholism, job instability, antisocial behavior, or psychiatric illness." Critics conceded that some of these criteria may be medically relevant, but worried that others incorporated unarticulated, undefended, and even indefensible criteria of "social worth," perhaps in violation of procedural and substantive standards of fairness.

As a result of the uncertainty surrounding cardiac transplantation, DHHS ordered a major National Heart Transplant Study, prepared by the Battelle Institute, to assess the "social consequences" before deciding whether to provide funds to pay for the operation. This study, which was submitted in 1984, determined that cardiac transplantation's success rates in length and quality of life, including rehabilitation for work, warranted viewing the procedure as nonexperimental. In 1986, the federal Task Force on Organ Transplantation also stressed the success of heart transplantation, noting that cyclosporine had recently improved the 1-year survival rate of heart transplant recipients to 75 to 85%. Because of such successes, the Massachusetts General Hospital reconsidered its decision and joined a consortium of Boston hospitals to provide cardiac transplantation, and the Health Care Financing Administration of DHHS in 1987 agreed to provide funds for a few heart transplants for Medicare-eligible patients at selected centers on the grounds that heart transplants are a medically reasonable and necessary service.

Some individuals can afford the $100,000 required for a heart transplant and the expensive follow-up care, and some insurance policies cover these procedures. However, many patients lack these resources and cannot meet the stringent Medicare criteria. As a result, the decision about whether society should pay for heart transplants has fallen to the states. The most publicized decision not to provide state Medicaid funds for heart transplants (and other transplants except for corneas and kidneys) occurred in Oregon. The Oregon legislature voted in 1987 to discontinue its Medicaid organ transplant coverage for an estimated 34 recipients over 2 years at an estimated cost of $2.2 million in order to provide basic health care for approximately 1,500 low-income children and pregnant women. The governor, Neil Goldschmidt, stated when he signed the bill into law: "We all hate it, but we can't walk away from this issue any more. It goes way beyond transplants. How can we spend every nickel in support of a few people when thousands never see a doctor or eat a decent meal?" The Oregon Senate president, John Kitzhaber, a physician, asked, "Is the human tragedy and the personal anguish of death from the lack of an organ transplant any greater than that of an infant dying in an intensive care unit from a preventable problem brought about by a lack of prenatal care?"

In addition to these debates about the so-called "green screen"—the criterion of ability to pay—patient selection criteria are still controversial, whether for admission to the waiting list or assignment of a particular organ. The supply of donated organs is limited. In 1988 there were 1,647 heart transplants, and in May 1989 there were 1,239 people on the waiting list of the United Network of Organ Sharing (UNOS), many of whom died before they could receive a heart (for figures on major organ transplants in United States, see the Appendix). Over the last few years UNOS has developed and further modified criteria for distributing hearts and other organs, considering such factors as urgency of medical need, probability of successful transplantation, and time on the waiting list. There is vigorous debate about how to make these factors operational (e.g., how many points to assign to each factor) and about the relevance of other factors, such as age, contribution of a person's lifestyle to the end-stage organ failure, and social network of support.

Perhaps because of unfair admission to waiting lists, patients receiving heart transplants tend to be white males over 45 years of age.[1]

I have several reasons for choosing to focus my presentation on this case study. First, organ transplantation is often taken as a paradigm and a test case in debates about fair access to health care. Careful examination of the debates regarding the allocation and distribution of organs for transplantation, including the relevance of ability to pay, can illuminate other debates about fairness in health care, even though, as we will see, organ transplantation may raise some unique issues. Second, much of my own experience in public policy in health care has centered on organ transplantation. I served for 2 years on the Board of Directors of the United Network for Organ Sharing (UNOS), which is the national organ procurement and transplantation network (OPTN), and in 1985–1986 I served as vice-chairman of the federal Task Force on Organ Transplantation. Both the Task Force and UNOS have helped to shape many of the public policies that now govern the distribution and allocation, as well as the procurement, of organs for transplantation.[2] The Task Force had the special responsibility of making "recommendations for assuring equitable access by patients to organ transplantation and for assuring the equitable allocation of donated organs among transplant centers and among patients medically qualified for an organ transplant."[3] (In this context I will construe "equity" as equivalent to "fairness," and I will sometimes use the term "justice" as equivalent to both of them.) Third, this case study involves the complex mixture of ethical, social, scientific, and medical factors that appear in hard choices in the allocation and delivery of health care. It is not always possible to distinguish or separate these factors and to identify one factor as *the* ethical factor.

SELECTION OF RECIPIENTS OF SCARCE ORGANS
FOR TRANSPLANTATION

The scarcity of organs for transplantation will probably remain a problem for the indefinite future; indeed, it is possible that the demand will always exceed the supply. Under these circumstances, there will be difficult questions regarding the procedural and substantive standards for patient selection. Who should choose recipients of donated organs and by what criteria?

Donated Organs as Public Resources

Why not simply let the physicians, nurses, and others involved in transplantation select patients? Why shouldn't selection be viewed as a medical decision to be made by the appropriate professionals? There are some important reasons for general public criteria of patient selection—criteria that are developed with input from the public and publicly stated and defended. Apart from special cases—for example, when living donors of kidneys designate a recipient or beneficiary—it can be argued that from a moral standpoint, donated organs belong to the public, to the community. This fundamental conviction undergirded the Task Force's deliberations and recommendations regarding fair access to organ transplantation: Donated organs should be viewed as scarce public resources to be used for the welfare of the community. Organ procurement and transplant teams receive donated organs as trustees and stewards for the community. Their dispositional authority over those organs should be limited and constrained.[4]

There is increasing demand that the public participate in formulating the criteria for patient selection in order to ensure that they are fair. In general, the evidence presented to the Task Force indicated that organ procurement and transplantation teams have usually made morally responsible decisions in the allocation and distribution of organs. However, some widely publicized exceptions generated public controversy and perhaps even reduced organ donations. The increasing demand for public participation in the formulation of criteria for the allocation and distribution of organs stems in part from the nature of the organ procurement system—it depends on voluntary gifts by individuals and families to the community. Indeed, there are important moral connections between policies of organ procurement and policies of organ distribution. On the one hand, it is obvious that the success of policies of organ procurement may reduce scarcity and hence obviate some of the difficulties of patient selection. On the other hand, distrust is a major reason for public reluctance to donate organs, and policies of procurement may be ineffective if policies of distribution are perceived by the public to be unfair and thus untrustworthy.[5] Hence public participation—for example, in UNOS—is important. As Jeffrey Prottas insists, "Organ allocation falls into the region of public decision making, not medical ethics and much less medical tradition."[6]

Morally Relevant and Irrelevant Characteristics

Justice not only involves public participation—a matter of fair process—but also substantive standards. "Justice" may be defined as rendering each person his or her due, and it includes both formal and material criteria. The formal criterion of justice is similar treatment for similar cases, while material criteria specify relevant similarities and dissimilarities among patients and thus determine how particular benefits and burdens will be distributed.[7] There is debate about the *moral relevance* and *moral weight* of various material criteria, such as need, merit, societal contribution, status, and ability to pay. Different theories of justice tend to accent different material criteria; however, some criteria may be acceptable in some areas of life but not in others.

A fundamental issue for organ transplantation is determining which material criteria are justifiable for the allocation and distribution of donated organs. Standards of justice permit rationing under conditions of scarcity, but they rule out selection criteria that are based on morally irrelevant characteristics, such as race or sex. The major debates focus on which characteristics of patients are morally relevant and which are morally irrelevant in the two stages of selection for organ transplantation: (1) formation of a waiting list, and (2) distribution of available organs to patients on the waiting list.

Admission to Waiting Lists

There is general agreement that the waiting list of candidates for transplantation should be determined primarily by medical criteria: the need for and the probability of benefitting from an organ transplant.[8] There is, of course, debate about whether these medical criteria should be defined broadly or narrowly (for example, how high should we set the standard for minimal efficacy?), about how to specify these criteria, about the relevance of several different factors to the determination of need and efficacy, and about which criteria should have priority in case of conflict.

Why are both need and probability of success important? They reflect *medical utility,* which requires the maximization of welfare among patients suffering from end-stage organ failure. Medical utility should not be confused with *social utility.*[9] Whereas social utility focuses on the value of salvageable patients for society, medical utility requires that organs be used as effectively and as efficiently as possible to benefit as many patients as possible. For example, if there is no reasonable chance that a transplant will be successful for a particular patient, it could even be unethical to put the patient in line to receive a scarce organ.

Efforts are being made through UNOS and elsewhere to develop fair policies of organ allocation and distribution, but it is more difficult to ensure equitable access to waiting lists for organ transplants. There is evidence that women, minorities, and low-income patients do not receive transplants at the same rates as white men with high incomes.[10] For example, in one study, females were approximately 30% less likely than males to receive a kidney transplant, black dialysis patients were only 55% as likely as whites to receive a cadaver transplant, and patients receiving dialysis in units in higher income areas had higher transplant rates.[11] The primary source of unequal access appears to be in the decisions about who will be admitted to the waiting list rather than the decisions about who will receive donated organs. However, more research will be required to determine the extent to which unequal access to kidney transplantation, for example, hinges on patient choices and legitimate medical factors rather than on physician sequestration of patients in dialysis units, physician failure to inform and refer some groups of patients, or physician bias in the selection of patients seeking admission to waiting lists.

UNOS Point System for Cadaveric Kidneys

Although UNOS has developed computerized point systems for the allocation of hearts, livers, and kidneys, I will use the point system for kidneys as the primary example because it has received the most attention and has undergone the most alterations in light of conflicting values. In October 1987, UNOS implemented a point system for cadaveric kidneys, based on a proposal by Thomas Starzl and colleagues.[12] This system required that cadaveric kidneys be offered to patients on the local waiting list (defined as either the individual transplant center recipient list or a shared list of recipients within a defined procurement area) in descending order, with the patient with the highest number of points receiving the highest priority. The original point system consisted of three major parameters: the degree of sensitization, reflected in panel reactive antibodies (PRA, 10 points maximum), time on the waiting list (10 points maximum), and HLA matching (12 points maximum), with some attention to logistics and urgency. Critics noted that the point values for time waiting and high PRA overrode all other point allocations so that the first patient to appear on the printout had high PRA levels, but poor HLA matches. And most of the requests for area variances involved PRA and antigen match.

After much discussion, in 1989 UNOS adopted a revised point system that stresses HLA matching because of evidence about its long-term impact on graft survival. This revised point system accords less weight to sensitization and to time on the waiting list, as well as to logistics and urgency. According to the UNOS policy statement, "for the national pool, the new allocation system will ensure optimal use of every cadaver kidney offered, since it will identify very well matched recipients. Highly sensitized patients will be chosen when excellent matches emerge. Kidneys will be shipped to highly sensitized patients generally only when negative crossmatches had [sic] been obtained at the donor center. Within each match category, fractions of a point acquired for waiting time will determine the order in which patients with the same match score would be listed."[13] Medical urgency status can be requested under some circumstances, but they are rare because dialysis is usually possible as a backup. The policy of mandatory sharing of zero antigen mismatches continues, and a payback policy has been adopted for centers receiving organs that had to be shared. ABO blood group matching will remain the same—blood group "O" kidneys may be transplanted only into blood group "O" patients except in the case of kidneys that are mandatorily shared because of HLA match; otherwise, "O" patients would be greatly disadvantaged because "O" organs are usable in other blood groups whereas "O" patients can use only "O" organs. (UNOS point systems for hearts and livers have also generated some controversy, as will be evident in the discussion that follows.[14])

Assessment of Point Systems for Allocation of Organs

How are these point systems to be assessed? I will first consider the value of computerized point systems in general and then the value of these particular point systems. Many of the supposed advantages and disadvantages of point systems for the allocation of organs hinge on their alleged *objectivity*. Even though the point system does not eliminate the individual physician's judgment—the art of medicine—regarding, for example, the final decision about the use of an organ for any particular patient, the point system does reduce the physician's discretion. For example, Thomas Starzl contends that "the effect of [his original] point system was to diminish judgmental factors in case selection, which in the past probably had operated to the disadvantage of 'undesirable' potential recipients, including older ones and possibly ethnic minorities."[15] Even though many concede that decisions have been affected by physicians' subjective biases—for example, in admission to waiting lists—many also note the importance of physicians being able to practice the art of medicine in view of the individual features of particular cases, such as predicting efficacy for a particular patient. Daniel Wikler contends that a computerized point system can systematize decision making by focusing on a full range of data and "can convince patients and the public that a routine, sound plan is in place," perhaps enhancing the perception of fairness in distribution or at least stimulating public discussion.[16] However, in focusing on objectivity, we must not forget that the selection of and assignment of weights (points) to these factors rest on values.

With the exception of time on the waiting list, the criteria used in the different point systems for kidneys are medical in the sense that they involve medical techniques used by medical personnel and arguably influence the likely success or failure of the transplant. However, even though these criteria are medical in these senses, they are not value-free or value-neutral.[17] The vigorous debate about how much weight each criterion should have is only in part technical and scientific (e.g., the impact of HLA matching); it is to a great extent ethical. In kidney transplantation, some factors, such as quality of antigen match and logistical score, focus on the chance of a successful outcome. In different ways both medical urgency and panel-reactive antibody focus on patient need; and time on the waiting list introduces a nonmedical factor, even though it may overlap with panel-reactive antibody because sensitized patients tend to wait longer for transplants. The points assigned to these various factors thus reflect value judgments about the relative importance of patient need, probability of success, and time of waiting—all factors stressed by the federal Task Force on Organ Transplantation.[18]

Medical Utility in Patient Selection

Both patient need for a transplant and the probability of a successful transplant reflect medical utility. Medical utility is not necessarily at odds with fairness, even though they may sometimes come into conflict. It is a fundamental mistake to suppose that "medical utility" and "fairness" are necessarily in tension so that if one is met, the other is infringed, and it is a fundamental mistake to suppose that "fairness" always dictates priority to queuing or randomization over "medical utility." Indeed, in some contexts determination of "medical utility" may be required by the principle of fairness. It may be "unfortunate" when one patient receives an organ over another because of "medical utility," but it is not necessarily "unfair." Appeals to "medical utility" in the distribution of organs do not necessarily violate the principle of equal concern and respect; judgments based on "medical utility" do not necessarily show disrespect and contempt that may be evident in judgments based on patients' comparative "social utility."[19] Furthermore, acceptance of "medical utility" does not commit one to utilitarianism as a foundational or substantive moral doctrine; "medical utility" can (and should) be accepted in any defensible deontological framework as well. Holding that a lexical or serial order of these criteria is impossible also does not entail utilitarianism. In addition, using a Rawlsian contract metaphor, we can argue that in a fair set of decision-making circumstances behind the veil of ignorance, patients not knowing their own medical conditions would choose criteria of "medical utility."[20] Such a hypothetical contract allegedly makes the distribution fair to potential recipients. Finally, others also argue that fairness to donors requires that organs be used effectively and efficiently.[21]

As already noted, judgments about medical need and probability of success are value laden. For example, there is debate about what will count as *success*—such as length of graft survival, length of patient survival, quality of life, rehabilitation—and about the factors that influence the *probability of success*. Some contraindications are well established, such as mismatched blood group or positive donor–recipient crossmatch. The revised UNOS point system for kidneys stresses tissue matching on medical utility grounds. It is also not unfair to use tissue matching, not only because of medical utility, but also because tissue matching functions as a form of the natural lottery, involving the randomness of the HLA match between available donors and recipients.[22] However, there is vigorous debate about the relative importance of tissue matching now that cyclosporine is available, and this technical debate influences judgments about the conditions under which kidneys should be shared outside the location where they are retrieved. For example, since cyclosporine is nephrotoxic, a retrieved kidney needs to be transplanted sooner than usual in order to increase the chances of successful transplantation.

Tissue matching needs ongoing scrutiny. First, in view of the scientific controversy, it is essential to see if tissue matching really makes a significant difference in the outcome of transplantation over time. Second, it is morally imperative to monitor the operation of the revised point system to make sure that tissue matching does not have unjustified discriminatory effects, for example, against blacks and other minorities. It appears that there may already be discrimination against blacks and other minorities in admission to waiting lists, and tissue matching may have discriminatory effects for some patients on the waiting list. For example, most organ donors are white; certain HLA phenotypes are different in white, black, and Hispanic populations; the identification of HLA phenotypes is less complete for blacks and Hispanics; nonwhites have a higher rate of end-stage renal disease; and nonwhite populations are disproportionately represented on dialysis lists.[23] In this context, Robert Veatch argues that "[i]f organs are to be allocated on the basis of degree of tissue match, the policy is, de facto, a whites-first policy."[24] Monitoring the operation of the current point system will provide evidence regarding discriminatory effects. If such discriminatory effects emerge, then it may be necessary to sacrifice some probability of success in order to take affirmative action to protect blacks and other minorities.

Sometimes there is a tension between urgency of need and probability of success. Robert Veatch contends that "a justice-based allocation . . . would demand that highest priority be given to medical need and length of time the patient has been in need."[25] Apparently some potential recipients would choose such criteria. For example, members of a Canadian transplant team have written: "When determining who will get a heart, it becomes a difficult ethical issue as to whether the patient with the better outcome or the individual with the greatest urgency should receive the heart. The patients themselves would opt for the patient with the greatest urgency and by and large that is the decision taken by the team. However, one is conscious of the fact that one may be affecting the overall success rate by making choices in favour of individual patient urgency rather than making them on the basis of success."[26]

Tensions between medical urgency and probability of success may vary greatly depending on the organ in question. For instance, there is debate in heart transplantation about the use of artificial hearts and other assist devices, in part because they have sometimes given patients priority for scarce donor hearts on the basis of medical need, even though their chances for success may be minimal. Critics such as George Annas charge that using the total artificial heart as a temporary bridge to transplantation does not save lives; it only changes the identities of those receiving heart transplants by giving very sick patients priority.[27] UNOS has recently revised its criteria for the allocation of hearts so that patients on mechanical assist devices will no longer receive priority over all other candidates in their area; under the new allocation system, patients who require inotropic agents and are in intensive care units will also be in the top priority group. This revision should remove any incentive for a physician to put a patient on an assist device in order to improve his or her chances of getting a heart transplant.[28]

To take another example, in liver transplantation the dominant practice has been to give the sickest patient the highest priority, but "medical utility" (and some would include cost-effectiveness) would appear to be served by placing the liver in the fittest patient and realizing the most medical benefit (at the lowest cost). Another reason for priority to those with a higher probability of benefit is that "as time goes on . . . the fitter patients become increasingly ill, their survivability on the waiting list declines, and their operative risk soars."[29] Nevertheless, as Olga Jonasson notes, there is clearly one case in which the sickest of all patients awaiting liver transplants is also the best candidate for successful transplantation: the young, previously healthy patient with fulminant acute liver failure.[30]

The category of medical urgency may not be as important when an artificial organ can be used as a backup (as dialysis can function for end-stage renal failure). However, some argue that medical urgency should include not only the immediate threat of death but also the likelihood of not receiving another organ because of presensitization, particularly because sensitized patients now constitute a hard core of the waiting lists for kidney transplants. The Task Force recommended that a highly sensitized patient who is predicted, on the basis of either a computer antibody analysis or an actual cross-match, to accept the transplant should be given priority over equivalently matched nonsensitized patients. And yet the success rates may be lower for sensitized patients than for nonsensitized patients.[31]

One problem is that medical urgency is a manipulable category, and it is reportedly abused at times by physicians eager to protect their patients by declaring them medically urgent in order to increase their chances for a transplant.[32] These reports are not implausible in light of studies indicating that physicians are willing to lie in order to promote their patients' welfare in the health care system, such as using a misleading category in order to enable the patient to have a diagnostic procedure covered by health insurance.[33]

In short, it is not at all clear that a general, a priori formulation of the appropriate relation between medical need and probability of success within medical utility is defensible, in part because of the variations in organ systems. Thus, the proposals may have to be organ specific, and variations can be expected in UNOS policies from one organ to another. Ongoing monitoring and assessment of current policies, with public input and with special attention to the proper use of the category of medical urgency, appear to be the most appropriate actions.

Time on the Waiting List

Many, including this writer, have argued that randomization or time on the waiting list is a fair way to allocate scarce life-saving resources under some circumstances. I developed my argument to this effect in 1970 when the debate was mainly about kidney dialysis.[34] At that time I argued that once the pool of medically eligible candidates has been determined, it is then fair to make the final selection by randomization or queuing. I believe that matters are somewhat different when the scarce medical resource is an organ that cannot be reused. Now I would argue that medical utility should also be used to determine which candidate should receive the organ, after the eligible candidates have been identified on grounds of medical utility. A major reason is not wasting the gift of life; the organ has been donated for effective use. Giving an organ to a patient who has a very limited chance of success, perhaps because of poor tissue match, increases the probability that he or she will then need another transplant for survival, further reducing the chances for others as well as for his or her own successful transplantation. (Retransplantation will be discussed below.) However, it is important to reject positions that rule out queuing or time on the waiting list as morally irrelevant. For example, Olga Jonasson argues that "length of time on the waiting list is the least fair, most easily manipulated, and most mindless of all methods of organ allocation," and Ruth Macklin argues that principle of "first come, first served" is inapplicable and even inequitable in the allocation of scarce medical resources because it ignores different medical needs and prognoses.[35]

By contrast to those positions, if two or more patients are equally good candidates for a particular organ according to the medical criteria of need and probability of success, their time on the waiting list may be the fairest way to make the final selection. This approach is similar to that recommended by the federal Task Force.[36] The original UNOS point system for kidneys gave more weight to time on the waiting list and also to sensitization, but since highly sensitized patients are likely to spend more time on the waiting list, they were, in effect, counted twice. Some would argue that such double counting is justifiable because of their difficulty of obtaining organs, while others would note that such patients may then receive priority over much better matched patients. Now time on the waiting list functions more as a tie-breaker in the allocation of kidneys in the UNOS point system.

Queuing is often favored because it appears to be objective and impersonal, but the justification of its use in patient selection depends on certain values (or principles), such as fair opportunity. However, practically and ethically, there are problems. It is not always easy to determine when a patient entered the waiting list; one way is the accession time on the UNOS list. But, as Jonasson notes, it is easy to manipulate this criterion, for example, by putting patients on the list before they become dialysis dependent.[37] In addition, it is important to note that the fairness of queuing (as well as of randomization) depends in part on background conditions. For example, some people may not seek care early because of limited financial resources and insurance; others may receive inadequate medical advice about how early to seek transplantation, etc.

Number of Previous Transplants

Retransplantation raises important issues of fairness and medical utility—for example, in cases of patients receiving three or four liver transplants. Between 1977 and 1981, 10,818 patients received 11,615 kidney transplants, with 10,063 patients receiving one transplant, 713 patients receiving two, and 42 patients receiving three or more.[38] The argument is sometimes made that fair access to scarce organs for transplantation should limit a patient to one transplant, but others resist this conclusion on the grounds that denying a transplant recipient another transplant is tantamount to abandonment. However, it is difficult to sustain the claim of abandonment if there are back up or alternative treatments, such as dialysis for end-stage renal disease. And from the standpoint of medical utility, it appears that the chances for successful transplantation decline somewhat after each transplant.[39]

Other Controversial Criteria

Several other criteria have been proposed for patient selection, and it is important to examine them carefully in order to make sure that they reflect medical utility, rather than social utility, and that they are not otherwise unfair. For example, as the case study noted, in 1980 former DHHS Secretary Patricia Harris withdrew the earlier tentative authorization for Medicare to cover some heart transplants in part because of her concern that some criteria for patient selection were more social than medical. Because judgments of social utility may masquerade as judgments of medical utility, it is essential that the criteria of patient selection be publicly developed and articulated as well as fairly applied. The public process is important to ensure that the criteria are based on medical utility, rather than on social utility, and also reflect both fairness and respect for persons. Several possible criteria are very controversial because they may function as guides either to medical utility or to social utility—for example, age, social network of support, life-style, and behavioral patterns.[40] One question is whether they can legitimately function as guides to medical utility without implying judgments of social utility and infringing principles of justice and respect for persons.

ABILITY TO PAY

So far I have examined issues of patient selection for organs for transplantation—both formation of the waiting list and selection to receive a particular organ—apart from questions of costs. Yet organ transplants are notoriously very expensive. (For the relevant figures, see the Appendix.) Our society has responded very differently to different organ transplant procedures. Through Medicare's End-Stage Renal Disease (ESRD) program, virtually everyone who needs a kidney transplant (or dialysis) is covered, while coverage for heart and liver transplantation is more spotty. Should ability to pay be accepted as a criterion? Should there be what has been called a "green screen" for access to organ transplantation? These are not questions that can be directly addressed by UNOS; they emerge on other levels for other social institutions, particularly the federal and state governments.

As part of its efforts to propose policies to ensure equitable access to organ transplantation, the federal Task Force on Organ Transplantation offered several arguments in favor of increasing societal funding for organ transplants—on the one hand, for immunosuppressive medications for organ transplants already funded (mainly kidneys), and, on the other hand, for extrarenal organ transplants not currently funded. The Task Force argued that coverage for immunosuppressive medications was important because, for example, wealth discrimination had reentered the ESRD program, which had been designed to eliminate distribution of artificial and transplanted kidneys according to ability to pay. Noting that approximately 25% of the transplant population (for all organs) lacked state or private coverage for immunosuppressive medications, especially cyclosporine, which was then estimated to cost approximately $5,000–7,000 a year, the Task Force "found evidence that inability to pay for immunosuppressive medications had been a factor in the initial selection of patients for transplantation" and that some transplant recipients had undergone nonmedically indicated—and potentially risky—changes in their medications because of the costs.[41] The Medicare coverage that was subsequently approved, in part in response to the Task Force report, was limited to 1 year after the transplant. Further study is needed to determine whether this limited coverage has reduced those problems.

Much of the Task Force's concern about fair access focused on extrarenal organs—hearts and livers—in view of the limited and uneven provision of funds for them. And, according to the Task Force, there are several arguments for a societal obligation, to be discharged by the federal government as a last resort, to provide funds for extrarenal transplants in order to ensure fair access.

One argument focuses on the *continuity* between extrarenal organ transplants and other medical procedures that are already covered, such as kidney transplants and dialysis. Appealing to the principle of consistency or universalizability, this argument accepts the precedential value of prior and current policy decisions. Still another premise in the argument is empirical—extrarenal transplants are comparable in efficacy and costs to procedures that are routinely covered. In response to worries about cost containment, defenders of public funding for organ transplantation hold that it is unfair to impose the major burden of cost containment on patients with end-stage organ failure who need transplants. The demands of cost containment should themselves be distributed equitably across categories of patients needing health care.[42]

A second argument focuses on the *distinctiveness or uniqueness* of organ transplantation, particularly the social practices of procurement that provide the organs for transplantation. This argument identifies an important moral connection between organ procurement, including organ donation, and organ distribution and allocation.[43] In its efforts to increase the supply of organs, our society requests donations of organs from people of all socioeconomic classes—for example, through presidential appeals for organ donations or, more recently, through state "required request" and "routine inquiry" statutes, which mandate that institutions inquire about an individual's or family's willingness to donate or even request such a donation. However, it is unfair and even exploitative for the society to ask people, rich and poor alike, to donate organs if access to donated organs will be determined by ability to pay rather than by medical need, probability of success, and time on the waiting list.[44]

A third and related argument builds on societal opposition to commercialization and commodificaton of human body parts, as expressed in various laws and policies. Federal legislation—as well as legislation in some states—prohibits individuals from transferring organs over which they have dispositional authority for valuable consideration.[45] In addition, various professional organizations involved in organ transplantation have taken a stand against the sale of organs for transplantation. It is difficult, according to this third argument, to distinguish (1) buying an organ for transplantation and then hiring a surgeon to perform the procedure from (2) purchasing an organ transplantation procedure that includes a (donated) organ as well as the surgeon's (and others') services.

These last two principled arguments may be combined with consequentialist arguments. There are legitimate worries about the impact of unequal access to organ transplants, based on inability to pay, on the system of organ procurement that includes gifts of organs from individuals and their families. As I noted earlier, there is substantial evidence that attitudes of distrust limit organ donation; this distrust appears to be directed at both organ procurement (e.g., the fear the potential donors will be declared dead prematurely) and organ distribution (e.g., the concern that potential transplant recipients from higher socioeconomic classes will receive priority).[46] Thus, it is not at all surprising that after Oregon decided to stop providing Medicaid funds for most organ transplants, "a boycott of organ donations was organized by some low-income people."[47]

A final argument is closely related to the first one, but, instead of building on what the society has already decided to do regarding other health care, it focuses on the federal government's obligation, at least as a last resort, to ensure fair access to health care, including organ transplantation, by removing financial barriers, if necessary. For example, this argument might appeal to what the President's Commission construed as society's obligation to provide equitable access to an adequate level of health care without excessive burdens.[48] (Even though this argument may appear to be independent of social practices, it may—and should—nevertheless appeal to principles and values embedded in those practices.) Whatever the foundation of the obligation, there will still be vigorous debate about what counts as an adequate level of health care and whether organ transplants qualify. And this debate moves us to questions of *macroallocation*. It is now standard to distinguish microallocation from macroallocation. For example, Engelhardt uses the term "macroallocation" to refer to "allocations among general categories of expenditures," and the term "microallocation" to refer to "choices among particular individuals as to whether they will be recipients of resources and in what amount."[49]

MACROALLOCATION DECISIONS

The question of microallocation is *who* will receive a particular scarce good; the questions of macroallocation focus on *how much* of a good will be made available, where financial resources can alter the availability of that good, such as organ transplants or AZT for AIDS patients. It is important to note that although macroallocation and microallocation are analytically distinct, they are significantly related. Obviously macroallocation decisions determine the extent of scarcity and the difficulty of patient selection by in part determining how much of a good will be made available in a society. If a particular technology or mode of health care is in limited supply, as is often the case, then there may be difficult microallocation decisions about who will receive this particular scarce good. But problems in microallocation may also have an impact on macroallocation decisions. For instance, it has been argued that the federal government decided to provide virtually universal funding for treatments for end-stage renal disease in part to eliminate the problem of patient selection for kidney dialysis and transplantation, that is, the problem of having health care professionals and committees explicitly determine who would live and who would die.[50]

At the lowest macroallocation level—the language of "levels" indicating the generality of the decision rather than its location in an institutional structure of decision making—it is necessary to decide which technologies and procedures should have priority in funding. In its concentration on organ transplantation, the federal Task Force did not address this issue, beyond noting that patients suffering from end-stage organ failure should not be made to bear the brunt of the society's efforts at cost containment. The decision about funding particular technologies has usually hinged on medical practice—what is reasonable and necessary medical care. However, there is widespread recognition that technology assessment directed toward societal funding of medical procedures should include other factors as well, beyond whether patients need and would probably benefit from the procedures. Often this debate is couched in terms of the distinction between experimental and nonexperimental procedures. However, this distinction is not merely scientific and technical, for it depends on such value questions as the balance between benefits and risks. Drawing a line between experimental and nonexperimental treatments is not exclusively scientific; it is also a matter of societal moral judgment.

Another macroallocation decision is presupposed by the determination of the fairness of funding particular medical technologies and procedures—which diseases should have priority in research and in care? Should end-stage organ failure have priority over other medical problems? And should heart disease have priority over arthritis or AIDS? One major shortcoming of the political process is the way some medical conditions attract attention while others fail to do so. Without question, end-stage organ failure has received attention far out of line with its overall significance in health care. An adequate explanation would include (but would not be limited to) the fact that organ transplantation involves the transfer of a body part from one human being to another, the former's death usually being a necessary condition for the latter's life.[51]

It is unclear how far it is possible to develop criteria for more defensible priorities. Proposals include such criteria as the pain and suffering various diseases involve, their costs, the chances for rehabilitation, the ages in life when they strike, and so forth. Probably our societal metaphor of medicine as war against disease and our sociocultural anxiety about death lead to an excessive concentration on killer diseases, such as forms of cancer, rather than on disabling diseases, such as stroke and arthritis, with their heavy demand for chronic care.[52] Nevertheless, it is possible to argue for priority for some diseases that are life-threatening because life is a condition for other values even if it is only a conditional value. End-stage organ failure may qualify under that rubric.

Still another more general level of macroallocation decisions concerns the relative priority to prevention and to critical care of rescue medicine, with heart transplants being a major example of critical care directed at the rescue of patients with end-stage heart failure. This level of macroallocation has been long debated. For example, Plato's *Republic* (403d–408c) recommends that society focus on prevention, especially through altering life-styles—no Attic pastry and no Corinthian girls! And it recommends that chronic care not be provided for those who cannot be rehabilitated to function in the polis. The ideal republic would provide medical care only for seasonal illnesses such as colds. Our society has a different allocational scheme—more to critical care and less to prevention. One question is whether it would be more effective and efficient to pursue survival and health by a different allocation scheme by putting more resources into prevention than into critical care. And, if such an allocational scheme would be more effective and efficient, the question is whether it would be fair.

This macroallocation decision should be subject to resolution in part through scientific and medical information about effectiveness in reducing morbidity and premature mortality. In some areas, however, we do not know enough to prevent diseases rather than treating them later. End-stage renal failure, for example, may result from several different causal factors. In some areas, the costs of prevention may be as great as (or even greater than) the costs of treatment.[53] And there are other reasons for society's tendency to concentrate on critical or rescue medicine. One reason is that critical care focuses on identified persons or lives, while prevention saves statistical lives.[54] These statistical lives may exist now, but we do not know which ones will be saved. In concentrating on identified lives, the society and health care professionals express the value of those lives and their own care and compassion in more dramatic ways than would be possible through prevention. However, there may be a tension between such symbolic actions and effective–efficient actions. This tension is also evident in society's allocation of more funds to try to rescue trapped miners than to try to prevent such disasters in the first place.

Another problem is that much prevention, including the prevention of heart disease and liver disease, may require the alteration of life-styles and behavioral patterns. Thus, the pursuit of a more effective and efficient preventive program may face moral and social limits set by the principles of respect for personal autonomy, liberty, and privacy, which, in general, protect individual life plans and risk budgets, unless agents are incompetent or their actions put others at risk. However, respect for autonomy is not absolute.[55] (There are also, as noted earlier, questions about whether the fact that a particular life-style is associated with end-stage organ failure is a morally relevant factor in the selection of patients for scarce organs for transplantation.)

Finally, we reach the most general macroallocation question, an answer to which is presupposed by all the others: How much of our society's budget should go into health and health care and how much into other social goods? Of course, some social goods other than medicine and health care contribute to health, but the conflict nevertheless has to be faced. It is not clear that it is wrong for the United Kingdom and many other countries to spend a lower proportion of their GNP on health care than the United States spends. Many would say that there are few, if any, right and wrong answers to this final general question. They hold that it is basically an aesthetic or a political question. It is *aesthetic* because a society can arrange its values in various ways to express its own identity. It is *political* because the answer emerges through the political process that can reflect the society's informal priorities. Even though survival and health are conditions for other values, they do not always take priority over those values.

However, there may be moral limits to such political and aesthetic decisions. If the principle of fairness (and social beneficence) supports the position that everyone in the society has a right to an adequate level or decent minimum of health care, then there must be at least enough in the society's budget to provide that minimum (with the government acting at least in the last resort). Various reports indicate that as many as 37 million Americans lack medical care—one-third of these are children—and that millions of others are underinsured. If we agree that there should be at least a decent minimum of health care, often expressed in the metaphor of a safety net, then debate will focus on determining that minimum and how that minimum itself should be allocated, for example, between prevention and rescue, between end-stage organ failure and other conditions, and between organ transplantation and other technologies. And it is important that the process of determining the minimum or adequate level of health care, as well as for making allocation decisions, be fair and perceived to be fair.[56]

CONCLUSION

In conclusion, I want to draw together several points and mention several others that grow out of this analysis. First, I have stressed the principle of fairness (equity or justice). This principle is not easy to specify or to apply, for there are vigorous disputes about its meaning (e.g., whether it includes medical utility) and about its weight (e.g., when it comes into conflict with other principles).

Second, fairness is not the only principle; there are others including beneficence, utility, and respect for personal autonomy. Fairness is not always in opposition to those principles, such as medical utility, as I argued in my proposals for a fair use of medical utility (medical need and probability of success) in the allocation and distribution of organs for transplantation. Even when there are conflicts, it is not possible to indicate in advance exactly which principle should have priority.[57]

Third, the implications of these various principles may differ for different questions and social institutions. In a closed system, such as Medicaid, where the trade-offs are clear and expansion of resources is not (at least immediately) possible, it may be entirely appropriate to make a careful cost-benefit analysis and decide not to provide funds for certain transplants, as occurred in such states as Oregon and Virginia. However, the arguments may be different in a more open system, such as the society as a whole, where it is not clear that choosing not to provide societal funds for extrarenal transplants would free those funds for basic health care for pregnant women and children, for example.[58]

Fourth, if we are asking a question about the fairness of providing or not providing funds for extrarenal transplants, it may be difficult to answer that question in an unfair system. If, as Norman Daniels argues, "our system is, in general, unjust,"[59] then it may be difficult to determine whether it would be just or unjust to press for and obtain funds for organ transplants or AZT or some other treatment. Which policy of allocation would be more likely to lead to a more just system? And, if neither would, which should be adopted as the morally preferable—perhaps because more just—policy within an unjust system?

Fifth, not only do our reflections about public policies occur within a particular sociopolitical context, but that context itself often changes over time. Thus, it may be appropriate to develop policies to salute some principles or values that have been neglected, or even overriden, in order to maintain their significance for the society over time.[60] There is no reason to suppose that within the range of ethically acceptable policies, only one should be implemented over time.

Finally, ethical theories, including theories of justice and fairness, may have limited applicability. Perhaps a satisfactory theory can identify a fair set of basic or other institutions with fair distributional patterns for health care and other goods. But such a theory may not satisfy conditions of feasibility. What then is the role for ethical theory? Perhaps the phrase "applied ethics"—the application of ethical theory—is not the most appropriate; perhaps the task for ethics is that of illuminating the ethical presuppositions and implications of the choices we have to make in the real world, in response to such questions as how organs should be distributed and allocated and whether organ transplants should receive societal funds. "Illumination" rather than "resolution" may be the main contribution of ethical theory, and it may take the form of "practical ethics" rather than "applied ethics."

APPENDIX

Major Organ Transplants in the United States

Year	Heart	Liver	Kidney
1975	23	9	3,730
. . . .	. . .	. . .	. . . .
1980	36	15	4,697
1981	62	26	4,883
1982	103	62	5,358
1983	172	164	6,112
1984	346	308	6,968
1985	719	602	7,695
1986	1,368	924	8,975
1987	1,512	1,182	8,967
1988	1,647	1,680	9,123
1989	1,673	2,160	8,890
Waiting lists, 5/89	1,239	760	14,949
Costs	$57,000–110,000	$135,000–238,000	$25,000–35,000

Other transplants in 1987:
Heart/lung—41 ($130,000–200,000)
Corneas—35,000 ($4,000–7,000)
Pancreas/islet cell—180 ($30,000–40,000)

Sources: The Task Force on Organ Transplantation, *Organ Transplantation: Issues and Recommendations* (April 1986); U.S. Department of Health and Human Services, Public Health Service, Health Resources and Services Administration, Division of Organ Transplantation, *Organ Transplantation: Q & A,* rev. October 1988; and data provided by the Division of Organ Transplantation and by the United Network for Organ Sharing (UNOS) Richmond, VA.

NOTES AND REFERENCES

1.   This case study is largely drawn from Case #33 in Tom L. Beauchamp and James F. Childress, *Principles of Biomedical Ethics,* 3rd ed. (New York: Oxford University Press, 1989), 446–449 (where complete references are given). References of particular importance include Roger W. Evans *et al., The National Heart Transplantation Study: Final Report* (Seattle: Battelle Human Affairs Research Center, 1984), and H. Gilbert Welch and Eric B. Larson, "Dealing with Limited Resources: The Oregon Decision to Curtail Funding for Organ Transplantation," *New England Journal of Medicine* 319 (1988): 171–173. See also Richard Rettig, "The Politics of Organ Transplantation: A Parable of Our Time," *Journal of Health*

Politics, Policy and Law 14 (Spring 1989): 191–227, and United States General Accounting Office, *Heart Transplants: Concerns about Cost, Access, and Availability of Donor Organs,* Report to the Chairman, Subcommittee on Health, Committee on Ways and Means, House of Representatives (Washington, DC: United States General Accounting Office, May, 1989).

2. See Task Force on Organ Transplantation, *Organ Transplantation: Issues and Recommendations* (Rockville, MD: Office of Organ Transplantation, Health Resource and Services Administration, U.S. Department of Health and Human Services, April 1986).

3. Public Law No. 98-507, "The National Organ Transplant Act."

4. See Task Force, *Organ Transplantation,* pp. 8–9, 85–86, *et passim.*

5. On the "moral connections" between procurement and distribution, see James F. Childress, "Some Moral Connections between Organ Procurement and Organ Distribution," *Journal of Contemporary Health Law and Policy* 3 (1987): 85–110.

6. Jeffrey M. Prottas, "Nonresident Aliens and Access to Organ Transplant," *Transplantation Proceedings* 21 (June 1989): 3428.

7. For a discussion of criteria of justice, see Beauchamp and Childress, *Principles of Biomedical Ethics,* Chap. 6.

8. Task Force, *Organ Transplantation,* Chaps. 4 and 5.

9. For the distinction between "medical utility" and "social utility," see James F. Childress, "Triage in Neonatal Intensive Care: The Limitations of a Metaphor," *Virginia Law Review* 69 (April 1983): 547–561.

10. See P. W. Eggers, "Effect of Transplantation on the Medicare End Stage Renal Disease Program," *New England Journal of Medicine* 318 (1989): 223–229; C. M. Kjellstrand, "Age, Sex, and Race Inequality in Renal Transplantation," *Archives of Internal Medicine* 148 (1988): 1305–1309; P. J. Held *et al.,* "Access to Kidney Transplantation: Has the United States Eliminated Income and Racial Differences?" *Archives of Internal Medicine,* 148 (December 1988): 2594–2600; and, for hearts, U.S. General Accounting Office, *Heart Transplants* (see note 1).

11. Held *et al.,* "Access to Kidney Transplantation." A draft report from the Office of the Inspector General indicates that blacks on kidney-transplant waiting lists have to wait almost twice as long as whites for a first transplant (13.9 compared with 7.6 months) and insists that this disparity cannot be explained solely by differences in "blood type, age, immunological and locational factors" because it remains even when these factors are controlled. See Inspector General's Report, Richard P. Kusserow, (Inspector General), U.S. Department of Health and Human Services, *The Distribution of Organs for Transplantation: Expectation and Practices,* OEI-01-89-00550 (draft report). The final report will appear after responses from various groups have been received.

12. See T. E. Starzl, T. R. Hakala, A. Tzakis *et al.,* "A Multifactorial System for Equitable Selection of Cadaver Kidney Recipients," *Journal of the American Medical Association* 257 (1987): 3073–3075.

13. UNOS, *Final Statement of Policy: UNOS Policy Regarding Utilization of the Point System for Cadaveric Kidney Allocation* (Richmond, VA: UNOS, April 4, 1989), which gives the history of the policy development as well as the current point

system. This document also provides an overview of the different stages and arguments involved in the policy formation.

14. See "Heart Allocation Policy," *UNOS Update* 5 (January 1989): 1–2.

15. T. E. Starzl, R. Shaprio, and L. Teperman, "The Point System for Organ Distribution," *Transplantation Proceedings* 21 (June 1989): 3434.

16. Daniel Wikler, "Equity, Efficacy, and the Point System for Transplant Recipient Selection," *Transplantation Proceedings* 21 (June 1989): 3437.

17. Dan Brock, "Ethical Issues in Recipient Selection for Organ Transplantation," in *Organ Substitution Technology: Ethical, Legal, and Public Policy Issues*, Deborah Mathieu, ed. (Boulder, CO: Westview Press, 1988), 86–99.

18. Task Force, *Organ Transplantation*.

19. See Daniel Wikler's argument in "Equity, Efficacy, and the Point System for Transplant Recipient Selection."

20. See *Ibid.*, and Martin Benjamin, "Value Conflicts in Organ Allocation," *Transplantation Proceedings* 21 (June 1989): 3378–3380. For further discussion, see the same issue, pp. 3413ff., particularly the comments by Ruth Macklin.

21. See Olga Jonasson, "Waiting in Line: Should Selected Patients Ever Be Moved Up?" *Transplantation Proceedings* 21 (June 1989): 3390–3394, and her comments in the discussion on p. 3413.

22. *Report of the Massachusetts Task Force on Organ Transplantation* (Boston, MA: Department of Public Health, October 1984).

23. Task Force, *Organ Transplantation*, Chaps. 4 and 5; Olga Jonasson, "Waiting in Line," p. 3393.

24. Robert M. Veatch, "Allocating Organs by Utilitarianism Is Seen as Favoring Whites over Blacks," *Kennedy Institute of Ethics Newsletter* 3 (July 1989): 1 and 3.

25. Robert M. Veatch, *Death, Dying and the Biological Revolution*, rev. ed. (New Haven, CT: Yale University Press, 1989), 210.

26. C. R. Stiller, F. N. McKenzie, and W. J. Jostuk, "Cardiac Transplantation: Ethical and Economic Issues," *Transplantation Today* 2 (February 1985): 24.

27. George Annas, "No Cheers for Temporary Artificial Hearts," *Hastings Center Report* 15 (October 1985), and "Death and the Magic Machine: Informed Consent to the Artificial Heart," in *Organ Substitution Technology*, ed. Deborah Mathieu, pp. 257–276.

28. See "Heart Allocation Policy."

29. Jonasson, "Waiting in Line," p. 3391.

30. *Ibid.*

31. Task Force, *Organ Transplantation*.

32. Comments by A. P. Monaco in roundtable discussion, *Transplantation Proceedings* 21 (June 1989): 3418.

33. Dennis H. Novack *et al.*, "Physicians' Attitudes Toward Using Deception to Resolve Difficult Ethical Problems," *Journal of the American Medical Association* 261 (May 26, 1989): 2980–2985.

34. James F. Childress, "Who Shall Live When Not All Can Live?" *Soundings* 53 (1970): 339–355. Contrast Childress, "Triage in Neonatal Intensive Care."

35. Jonasson, "Waiting in Line," p. 3392; Ruth Macklin, "Comment: Should Selected Patients Ever Be Moved Up?" *Transplantation Proceedings* 21 (June 1989):

3397. At least Jonasson's statement (and perhaps also Macklin's statement) can be construed as an objection to the *dominance* but not necessarily to the *relevance* of queuing, *ceteris paribus*.

36. See Task Force, *Organ Transplantation*, Chap. 5. Contrast *Report of the Massachusetts Task Force on Organ Transplantation*.

37. Jonasson, "Waiting in Line," p. 3393.

38. Task Force, *Organ Transplantation*, p. 90, drawn from Department of Health and Human Services, Office of Organ Transplantation, *Organ Transplantation Background Information*, February 1985.

39. See John Robertson, "Patient Selection for Organ Transplantation: Age, Incarceration, Family Support, and Other Social Factors," *Transplantation Proceedings* 21 (June 1989): 3401; A. P. Monaco, "Comment: A Transplant Surgeon's Views on Social Factors in Organ Transplantation," *Transplantation Proceedings* 21 (June 1989): 3406.

40. For a fuller discussion of some of these criteria, see James F. Childress, "Ethical Criteria for Procuring and Distributing Organs for Transplantation," *Journal of Health Politics, Policy and Law* 14 (1989): 87–113, reprinted in *Organ Transplantation Policy: Issues and Prospects*, James F. Blumstein and Frank A. Sloan, eds. (Durham, NC: Duke University Press, 1989), 87–113.

41. See Task Force on Organ Transplantation, *Report to the Secretary on Immunosuppressive Therapies* (Washington, DC: U.S. Department of Health and Human Services, October 1985), 1–3.

42. See Task Force, *Organ Transplantation*, Chap. 5.

43. *Ibid.*, Childress, "Ethical Criteria for Procuring and Distributing Organs for Transplantation."

44. Contrast Norman Daniels, "Comment: Ability to Pay and Access to Transplantation," *Transplantation Proceedings* 21 (June 1989): 3434.

45. See PL 98-507; see also Susan Denise, "Regulating the Sale of Human Organs," *Virginia Law Review* 71 (September 1985): 1015–1038.

46. See Childress, "Some Moral Connections."

47. H. G. Welch and E. B. Larson, "Dealing with Limited Resources," pp. 171–73.

48. President's Commission for the Study of Ethical Problems in Medicine and Biomedical and Behavioral Research, *Securing Access to Health Care* Vol. 1 (Washington, DC: U.S. Government Printing Office, 1983), Intro. and Chap. 1.

49. H. Tristram Engelhardt, Jr., *Foundations of Bioethics* (New York: Oxford University Press, 1986), 369, fn. 7.

50. Roger Evans, "Money Matters: Should Ability to Pay Ever Be a Consideration in Gaining Access to Transplantation?" *Transplantation Proceedings* 21 (June 1989): 3423; see Roger W. Evans, Christopher R. Blagg, and Fred A. Bryan, Jr., "Implications for Health Policy: A Social and Demographic Profile of Hemodialysis Patients in the United States," *Journal of the American Medical Association* 245 (1981): 478–491.

51. For a valuable interpretation of other issues, see Rettig, "The Politics of Organ Transplantation: A Parable of Our Time."

52. James F. Childress, "Ensuring Fairness, Respect, and Care for the Elderly," *Hastings Center Report* 14 (October 1984), 27–31.

53.   Louise Russell, *Is Prevention Better Than the Cure?* (Washington, DC: Brookings Institution, 1986).

54.   Thomas Schelling, "The Life You Save May Be Your Own," in *Problems in Public Expenditure Analysis,* Samuel B. Chase, Jr., ed. (Washington, DC: Brookings Institution, 1966), 127–166.

55.   James F. Childress, "The Place of Autonomy in Bioethics," *Hastings Center Report* 20 (January/February, 1990): 12–17. See also Childress, *Who Should Decide? Paternalism in Health Care* (New York: Oxford University Press, 1982).

56.   President's Commission, *Securing Access to Health Care.* For a fuller discussion of these macroallocation questions, see James F. Childress, *Priorities in Biomedical Ethics* (Philadelphia, PA: The Westminster Press, 1981), Chap. 4.

57.   Beauchamp and Childress, *Principles of Biomedical Ethics.*

58.   Norman Daniels, "Why Saying No to Patients in the United States Is So Hard: Cost Containment, Justice, and Provider Autonomy," *New England Journal of Medicine* 314 (1986): 1381–1383.

59.   Norman Daniels, "Comment: Ability to Pay and Access to Transplantation," p. 3424. For a fuller presentation of his position, see Daniels, *Just Health Care* (Cambridge, England: Cambridge University Press, 1985), which has greatly influenced these concluding remarks.

60.   Guido Calabresi and Philip Bobbitt, *Tragic Choices* (New York: Norton, 1977).

12

Equality, Justice, and Rightness in Allocating Health Care: A Response to James Childress

Robert M. Veatch

James Childress has given us a carefully reasoned and generally plausible account of an ethics of allocating resources and its implications for organ transplantation, one that reflects a moral theory far more subtle than a simple strategy of maximizing good consequences from the scarce health care resources we have available. He shows that the decisions made about ethical theory make a difference in how people will get treated by the health care system. Rather modest changes in the theory, however, can have important implications for decisions such as who should get scarce organs for transplantation.

I would like to suggest some places where some of these small changes in the general theory would be plausible and then comment on how that has forced me in my role as a member of the Washington Regional Transplant Consortium to vote for a different kidney allocation formula.

Childress and I agree that justice or fairness is one among several right-making principles for moral action. This implies that it is theoretically possible that, depending on one's formula for resolving conflict among ethical principles, a policy that is just or fair may turn out not to be exactly the policy that is ethically right, all things considered. Before tackling the question of the correct formula for resolving such conflict among principles, about which Childress and I differ on certain particulars, it is going to be necessary to clarify exactly what we mean by justice. Then I will try to reveal why this makes me opt for a somewhat different strategy for allocating kidneys than Childress appears to favor. I will close with some comments on how justice ought to relate to the other moral principles for allocating kidneys or any other scarce health resource.

THE PRINCIPLE OF JUSTICE

Deciding what is just or fair entails understanding whether there is a moral right-making characteristic of actions or policies or practices that is independent of the other usual considerations we take into account in deciding about right conduct. In particular, is the right allocation simply a matter of spreading resources around so that they produce the greatest amount of good in aggregate or so that people are free to act autonomously in using their private property; or is there some unique and independent consideration separate from these factors that pulls on us in deciding who should get a kidney or a scarce hospital bed or Medicare dollar?

Many ethical traditions have recognized that there is a moral principle independent of utility that bears on how resources should be distributed. They variously hold that there is a natural law, a law created by God, or that reason requires that one thing to consider in allocating resources is that they be distributed justly. One approach that permits some convergence of these disparate views is to ask what reasonable people would recognize as just if they had general knowledge of the facts of nature and human psychology, but no knowledge of their particular interests or needs. This approach does not necessarily require us to agree on why people under such circumstances would agree. Some might say they would agree because there is a preexisting moral law, others because reason would require it, or because it is a prudent way to protect self-interest. Regardless, there seems to be considerable convergence that, at least in certain circumstances, justice has something to do with an allocation that is not based solely on getting as much total or average utility out of the resources being allocated. Our sense of justice has something to do with recognizing the fundamental equality of persons. Although the argument cannot here be developed in detail, virtually all the ethical traditions participating in the current discussion recognize that the principle of justice creates a presumption in favor of equality. In my view, people under the circumstances I have described would agree that one right-making characteristic of an allocation practice would be that it gives people an opportunity for equality of well-being. This is what I shall refer to as the egalitarian principle of justice. Recall that whether it is right, on balance, to give people such an opportunity for equality of well-being will have to be settled later.

The only major variant on this formulation outside the utilitarian tradition is the Rawlsian maximin formula that commits society to practices that distribute goods—at least primary goods—equally except in cases in which everyone, especially the least well-off groups, would be benefited by unequal distributions. For purposes of health care allocation policies, the difference is minimal. The underlying difference, however, may be important. What is at stake is whether people's sense of justice (or God's sense of justice for those theologically inclined) includes an innate preference for people to be equal in their well-being, or whether equality is simply a device for maximizing individual well-being that should be waived when necessary for increasing the well-being of the least well-off. Rawls cannot imagine why anyone would find equality inherently preferable. He can only attribute a choice in favor of equality as resulting from envy. Surely, however, some relatively well-off persons have some inclination in favor of equality that is not based on envy. It is my interpretation that the pure principle of justice rests simply on our awareness that morality includes opportunities for equality as one of its right-making characteristics. If so, abandonment of equality when it is beneficial for the least well-off rests not on our sense of justice, but on some other moral consideration, something I will take up when we discuss the relation of justice to rightness.

This egalitarian principle of justice insists only on opportunities for equality of well-being. Thus an important and complex problem arises when people have such an opportunity but squander it with voluntary, risky life-style choices. In theory I see no reason why justice requires using scarce medical resources to treat medical needs resulting from such voluntary choices. Of course, other reasons may require covering such needs—the fact that it would be offensive to society to turn people needing such care away or terribly difficult to determine which needs were the result of truly voluntary choices. That does not imply, however, that justice is what requires providing such coverage. Furthermore, if we could develop a strategy to get voluntary risk takers to pay for their own care, it would be ethical to do so; in fact, justice would seem to require it. Thus, a health fee on smoking, alcohol consumption, skiing, and any other health risky behaviors deemed voluntary would be required by justice. The fee would not be designed to be a paternalistic deterrent. It would be calculated simply to reimburse the health system for the costs involved in providing care.

A second problem with the egalitarian principle of justice is that it requires opportunities for equality of well-being, not equality of health status. Thus, in theory it would be perfectly just for a health care system to permit two groups to have very unequal health status, provided the losing group was adequately compensated by advantages in other spheres of well-being. This means that, in theory, any discussion of justice in health policy has to take into account that unequal health can be compatible with the principle of justice.

As a practical matter, however, health is a unique entity, and in social organization it is quite separate from other spheres of well-being. In all other spheres of well-being (education being the exception), needs are distributed more or less equally. In health (and education), resources needed to approach equality are very unequal. Moreover, health care practices are administered as a more or less independent institution. Thus a good practical argument can be made that, in health policy, we should strive for opportunities for equality of health insofar as this is possible, leaving other social practices to deal with the best strategy for providing equality opportunities in other spheres of life. Thus, for practical purposes I will focus on justice in health care as requiring opportunities for equality of health. In doing so, I hold open the theoretical possibility that people should be able to trade their health resources for goods in other spheres. If such a practice were permitted, those making the trades would still have had the opportunity for equality of health.

There is one remaining theoretical problem. People evaluate purported benefits very differently. A ventilator providing support for a permanently vegetative patient may be perceived as of no benefit by most of us, while to some minority groups—some Orthodox Jews, for example—maintenance of permanently vegetative life may be a great good because life created by God is sacred regardless of consciousness. That is to say there is inherently subjective variation in what counts as a good. In spheres other than health care, we can resolve this matter rather easily by striving to distribute primary goods equally, letting people do their own allocating on the presumption that the result will be approximate equality of well-being or at least opportunities for it.

In health care, however, that clearly will not work. We simply must introduce a concept of objective well-being in the health sphere. People should have no moral claim of justice to a health resource—Laetrile, for example—simply because they believe it will increase their opportunity for well-being. Society will have to tackle the very difficult problem of determining what will be taken as contributing to objective rather than subjective well-being. We should not underestimate the difficulty or the importance of this task. Especially when we recognize that these judgments cannot be based on medical science and must rest on fundamental theological and metaphysical beliefs about what counts as a benefit, our society will have to confront a very difficult set of decisions in deciding how to promote opportunities for objective well-being in the health care sphere.

JUSTICE IN ALLOCATING ORGANS FOR TRANSPLANT

This brings us to the question of what would count as a just practice for allocation of kidneys or other organs for transplant. We should realize at this point that the just allocation is not necessarily the allocation that will produce the most benefit. In some cases, because of decreasing marginal utility, we find ourselves in the fortunate position that arranging resources so as to produce greater equality will also maximize the aggregate amount of good that is done. Transplantation, however, is one of many areas in health care where often a policy of giving resources to the worst-off group will be terribly inefficient in producing good because the worst off are so sick that large resource commitments do relatively little good. Thus we will have to decide not only what is just, but also whether the right course is based on producing justice, good health outcomes, or some combination thereof.

Childress is surely correct in dissociating justice from social utility. Even if considering the social usefulness of potential transplant recipients is a reasonable way of figuring out how to do the most good with organs, it is not the way to promote justice. He is also on the right track when he warns that medical criteria are not value free. Not only that, medical criteria may turn out to be surrogates for social criteria. Persons of lower social classes do more poorly medically. They lack the education, social support network, and resources to follow regimens necessary for the complex care following transplant. Physicians have correctly argued that patients were poor medical risks for transplant because of their fragile social environments. Appeals to medical criteria may simply be social criteria in disguise.

Childress goes on, however, to make a dangerously confusing claim. He says (p. 187) that "both patient need . . . and probability of successful transplantation reflect medical utility." It is particularly misleading, if not wrong, to say that "'medical utility' may be a criterion of fairness." I am not sure what this means, but, if I understand, I think this is simply wrong.

I take the criterion of medical utility to be that an individual has a moral claim to a transplant to the extent that it is predictable that a medical good will come from transplanting the organ to that individual. There is a great deal of room for dispute about what counts as a medical good, but that will not be critical here. We are talking about the prediction of the goods of years of life added or suffering and incapacity alleviated.

It should be conceded that allocating organs on the basis of medical utility may also happen to contribute to opportunities for equality of medical well-being, but that is surely an accident, not the result of striving for maximizing medical utility. Contrary to Childress, appeals to "medical utility" in the distribution of organs do necessarily violate the principle of equal concern and respect. The least well-off are not given equal respect; it is only luck if they happen to get the most medical utility from an organ. Often that will not be the case. Childress is correct that medical utility might be accepted in a deontological framework, but only to the extent that it incorporates some ethical principle other than justice. Some deontological frameworks do this. But it is a mistake not to recognize that, in such cases, the incorporation or medical utility takes place in spite of its prima facie violation of the justice principle. Only when we go on to examine the relation between justice and rightness will we be able to know if this is acceptable.

The UNOS point systems for allocating kidneys provide a perfect test case for practical application of one's understanding of justice in health resource allocation. As Childress describes, the original UNOS point system gave points for various factors including HLA matching, waiting time, panel reactive antibodies (PRA), logistics, and urgency. Although what follows will be somewhat of an oversimplification, it is within reason to attribute the various points in the formula to either medical utility or justice considerations. The 12-point maximum assigned to HLA were clearly points for the purpose of promoting medical utility. The degree of HLA match predicts the likelihood of a successful graft. On the other hand, the other points seem to be included as a way of giving transplant candidates a more equal chance of getting an organ even though the factors represented by the points generally have nothing to do with predicting medically good result. For example, the 10 points that could have been assigned for urgency surely have nothing to do with whether the transplant candidate would do well; to the contrary, the more urgent the transplant, the worse off the patient and the greater likelihood of a poor outcome. Likewise, points were included for PRA because persons with high PRA are more unlikely to have another chance to get an organ that is usable. Time on the waiting list is an indirect measure of how difficult it is for a person to be matched successfully. Thus persons with O blood group, high PRA, and antigens that are difficult to match are likely to be on the list a longer time and, if a suitable organ becomes available, they can be said to have greater need, not only because they have been waiting longer, but because they are less likely to get another chance.[1]

Still oversimplifying, one can say that the original Starzl formula used about one-fourth of its points (12 of 48) as a measure of medical utility and three-fourths as a measure of fairness or justice. It was thus not perfectly just, but gave justice considerable weight.

It should be pointed out how arbitrary this allocation was. Based on the original example in the Starzl proposal, if only antigen matching had been considered half as important, urgency twice as important, and waiting time scores calculated in proportion to length of wait, then the patient who scored the lowest would have moved to the top of the list. Nevertheless, the Starzl formula can be said to be approximately three-fourths committed to justice. Would that the same could be said for other governmental programs.

The real problem has arisen with the recently revised point system. Clinicians, typically being committed to medical efficiency even at the expense of justice, had protested that the Starzl formula was paying too much attention to need and not enough to medical utility. The result was a radical shift in the direction of antigen matching, the measure that is included because of the widespread belief that antigen matching increases probability of successful grafts. Now points included for medical utility have risen to approximately two-thirds of the total. Those whose need is great and who have a substantial chance to benefit from an organ will have a much harder time getting the organ. This is thought acceptable because they have somewhat less chance of benefit than others who get a large number of points for antigen matching.

One problem with this is that, contrary to Childress's claim (p. 188), likelihood of a good antigen match is far from random. Members of certain social groups are known to be statistically harder to match with an organ with a good chance of success. The losing groups strikingly are often those who are oppressed in other social allocations. Blacks and Hispanics, for example, are more likely to have antigens that are hard to match. Unidentifiable antigens are more frequent in these populations. For those for whom all six antigens cannot be identified, it is impossible to have a perfect match with a donor.[2]

Thus the point system is rigged so that blacks and Hispanics are known in advance to be at risk for not being able to get points. Likewise, women are known to have higher risk for panel-reactive antibodies. Although those with high PRA levels get points when they are matched with a suitable organ, those points can still be offset by the points assigned to others for a good tissue match, leaving the high PRA patient waiting in line even though possibly another suitable organ may never come along. Other groups known to be in need because they are difficult to match are those in the O blood group. If justice requires arranging social practices such as organ allocation systems so as to give people an equal opportunity, then the new (Terasaki) point system is far more unjust even than the original Starzl system. It is two-third rigged against justice, while the Starzl system is three-fourths justice-oriented.

Let me be very clear that I am not objecting in principle to the use of point systems for making allocation decisions. I agree that they provide at least some semblance of objectivity. Moreover, they give us a concrete formula for understanding how we are relating utility and justice. In the case of the new formula for kidneys, however, we are purposely demoting concerns for justice. We are making decisions that are known to work (statistically) against blacks, Hispanics, women, and others who are hard to match. Although to my knowledge the data are not available, it seems reasonable that the system will work against any who are in genetic groups distant from those that dominate the donor pool. It is likely, for example, that Jews, to the extent they reflect an atypical genetic endowment, will be hard to match. At the very least we should say of such an arrangement that we are sacrificing justice for medical utility. Whether that is ethically acceptable will have to be determined when we decide what the relation of justice to other ethical principles, such as utility or social beneficence, should be.

Before taking up that question, I want to use the kidney allocation formula to reveal how other, newer controversies about the theory of justice can be converted into the argument over points. We are in the early stages of an important debate over how age should affect what we consider to be a just allocation. It is easy to see how age would be taken into account by a utilitarian. Age is not only a predictor that a medical intervention will be more difficult, it is also evidence that the benefit of the intervention will last a shorter time. These considerations are not relevant, however, to the question of justice. Some committed to an egalitarian principle of justice would say that justice requires that age be ignored in deciding how resources should be allocated. Two people in equal need would get the same number of points in a kidney allocation regardless of the fact that one was 70 and the other 30 years of age.

There is a more complex interpretation of the principle of justice, however. It is true that if we view the question of who is worst-off at the moment in time when the kidney is needed, the 30-year-old and the 70-year-old could be said to be equally needy. They will both die (or need dialysis) without the organ. I refer to this as the "moment in time" perspective in assessing who is worst-off.

There is another perspective, however. I call it the "over-a-lifetime" perspective. It suggests that justice requires opportunity for equality of well-being over a lifetime. Another commentator has recently referred to this as the "complete lives" view of equality. From this perspective, the 30-year-old and the 70-year-old needing a kidney transplant are very different. The 70-year-old has had 40 more years. At the level of social policy we can only assume that these years were typical; they were at least years worth living. (To the extent that they were miserable years, that is a matter for other aspects of social policy to correct. I have argued that health care should for practical reasons be viewed as a separate practice.) From this over-a-lifetime perspective, the 70-year-old is much better off, and the 30-year-old has a stronger claim of justice to the kidney.

A point system could take this into account. It could assign points taking age into account. Daniel Callahan in *Setting Limits* has argued that social practices should recognize that some lives are complete and that, ethically, health resources for high-technology interventions should go to younger persons. He would, reasonably, assign a large number of points to anyone under his age cutoff and no points to those over it.

I do not accept the notion of a natural life span and the corollary that persons who have completed their life span have a radically different claim to health resources. Rather I hold that, from the over-a-lifetime perspective, the younger a person is, the fewer years of well-being he has enjoyed. This is a gradual variation, however. I would favor adding points to the allocation formula that are inversely proportional to age. I would assign points according to the formula:

$$\frac{1}{\text{age}} \times C$$

where C is a constant indicating how important age should be in comparison with other factors in the formula. Thus a 30-year-old would get twice as many points as a 60-year-old based on age consideration. A centenarian would get almost no points; an infant would get high weight because he has had almost no chance for well-being in life.

This intuition explains one reason why we are more eager to fund pediatric liver transplants than those for adults. (There are obviously other, less ethical, reasons.)

JUSTICE AND RIGHT ALLOCATION

This leads me to the conclusion that justice requires allocating health resources so as to produce opportunity for equality of health insofar as possible. To the extent that Childress incorporates other considerations, such as medical utility, we are in disagreement. I am particularly distressed when he says, apparently conveying what is just or fair, that "macroallocation decision[s] should be subject to resolution in part through scientific and medical information about effectiveness and efficiency in reducing morbidity and premature mortality" (p. 197). That is a formula that invites sacrificing fairness to the altar of aggregate efficient production of utility.

Still, I have admitted, as he has, that justice or fairness is not the only ethical consideration. There are other principles that could come into play in deciding what is the right allocation of scarce health resources. Some of these considerations are based on other principles that are deontological in character, that is, they do not focus directly on the production of good consequences. For example, it is conceivable that some scarce resources have been promised to individuals who do not have claims of justice to them. I am open, as apparently Childress is, to the necessity of balancing such competing moral principles as justice or autonomy or the duty to avoid killing.

The real controversy, however, is not over these principles, but rather over the conflict between justice and utility or social beneficence.[3] Childress says that "It is not possible to indicate in advance exactly which principle should have priority" (p. 199). Elsewhere, he has supported an approach that would balance competing claims. I want to go on record that I oppose this strategy as being terribly dangerous and contrary to our common moral sense.

First, note a double danger. Childress has already incorporated considerations of medical utility into his formulation of what is just or fair. He now tells us that justice or fairness will have to be further diluted by being balanced or prioritized with other principles, including utility or beneficence. If utility counts for half (or two-thirds in the new kidney formula) of what it means to be just or fair and then on top of that one must balance the fair course of action with the one that is called for by the principle of utility or beneficence, there is very little left of a commitment to equality of well-being. It is doubly diluted.

Even if Childress were to follow me in limiting justice to opportunity for equality of well-being, his approach of reconciling the claims of justice with those of utility would still be dangerous. It is a position that commits one logically to the view that in some cases if there is enough utility, the rights of individuals can always be sacrificed. In this case the right being sacrificed is an entitlement right, the right to the resources needed to have an opportunity for equality of well-being insofar as possible. In other cases the right may be a liberty right, such as the right to refuse medical treatment or refuse to be an unwilling subject of medical research. If justice and autonomy can be traded off against utility, one is logically committed to the position that, if enough good would be done, an individual can be sacrificed against his will to the aggregate good. That is a view I reject. It is a view the Judeo-Christian tradition rejects. It is a view that a liberal democratic society rejects. In particular, we are committed to the view that no amount of social good would justify coercing individuals to be subjects to Nazi-like medical experiments against their will. The only way one can remain committed in principle to that position is to acknowledge that no amount of beneficence or social utility can override the moral claims grounded in the nonconsequentialist principles such as autonomy or justice. In the example we are pursuing, no amount of medical utility should permit one to override the claim of justice that would lead to a policy of allocating scarce medical resources such as kidneys on the basis of who is worst-off.

This position is probably viewed by many, including Childress, as extreme. It is often challenged by what I call the infinite demand (or bottomless pit) argument. It is said that as soon as we come up against someone with an incurable medical need serious enough to classify the individual as among the worst-off, that person will command in the name of justice all society's resources. That would leave others destitute, which seems absurd.

The infinite demand problem is a serious one for an egalitarian, but there is a plausible response. First, all that is called for is opportunity for equality as far as possible. The principle does not call for using resources that will do no good for the least well-off. We do not need to give a kidney to someone dying of cancer. Assuming someone in a permanent vegetative state gets no objective benefit from medical treatment, we do not need to give a PVS patient a kidney.

Second, under the principle of autonomy, persons retain the right to refuse treatment. A person with a terrible incurable illness may find it appropriate to refuse treatment to let the dying process continue. He would not find the use of resources on his behalf beneficial.

Third, if literally all the world's resources went to someone medically incurable, eventually others would be even worse-off. They would become the ones with claims of justice. Although this is a limit at the extreme, it is a limit.

Fourth, I have acknowledged that other nonconsequentialist principles legitimately conflict with justice. If resources have been promised to others, they do not necessarily go to those who have claims of justice. Likewise, persons who are legitimate owners of resources may have autonomy rights that limit the use of resources for the least well-off. Also, the autonomy of the least well-off may lead them to yielding their claims of justice either because they are altruistic or because, as in the Rawlsian maximin case, they find it is in their interests to surrender their claims to equality. Contrary to Rawls, however, I describe this as waiving justice, not allocating in the name of justice. Moreover, in my formula it is only the least well-off who have the authority to waive the claims of justice. It is not something that rationality requires and therefore can be argued by anyone in the social system.

All of these taken together lead me to the confident conclusion that the bottomless pit problem is not an insurmountable one. If others, including Childress, do not agree, then they are forced to retreat to the dangerous territory where justice gets balanced against utility. That, however, is a terrible position to be in. I prefer to avoid it by never permitting mere utility to offset nonconsequentialist ethical considerations such as justice.

Even if such a balancing gamble is taken, however, it is still crucial to keep it separate from our conclusions about what is fair or just. If we have to incorporate points for HLA matching in our kidney allocation formula, let us at the very least state as clearly as possible that we are not doing it in the name of what is just or fair. Rather we are sacrificing justice in order to make the system more efficient or utility maximizing.

NOTES AND REFERENCES

1.   It is probably fair to point out that since high PRA also contributes to length of time on the waiting list, it may be double-counted in the formula.

2.   Technically, the points are assigned on the basis of mismatches. Still, if the donor organ has six identified antigens, then a recipient for whom only five antigens can be identified is said to have a mismatch for at least one of the donor's antigens. The maximum number of points is thus reduced accordingly.

3.   I will use the two interchangeably. Some would attempt to distinguish between beneficence and nonmaleficence and then determine a formula for relating the two. That is an interesting issue, about which Childress and I may disagree, but it is not crucial in this context.

III
DRAWING GUIDANCE FROM
OUR TRADITIONS

13

How to Draw Guidance from a Heritage: Jewish Approaches to Mortal Choices

David H. Ellenson

The progress made by medical science over the last half century has been astounding. In the area of therapeutic medicine alone, developments have been nothing short of miraculous. Heart transplants give life to people who otherwise would have died. Artificial insemination by a donor (A.I.D.) and *in vitro* fertilization offer infertile couples the possibility of conception and birth. Advances in genetic research raise the prospect that potentially fatal diseases or physical defects might be eliminated while the embryo is still *in utero*. Life support systems are now capable of maintaining the respiratory and circulatory functions of terminally ill patients indefinitely, while the invention of the electroencephalogram (EEG), combined with radionuclide cerebral angiography at the patient's bedside, permits doctors to confirm that irreversible, total brain death has occurred. These are among the almost countless advances made by medical researchers in our day.

Each of these discoveries, in addition to others not enumerated here, has presented doctors, nurses, patients, their families, and society with serious and often excruciating moral dilemmas. Are organs taken from animals permissible for use in human beings? Does A.I.D. constitute adultery? What does *in vitro* fertilization say about the meaning of parenthood? Does genetic engineering represent an unwarranted act of hubris on the part of human beings? If life is being maintained artificially through the use of a machine, is it morally acceptable to terminate life supports that will allow the patient to die? If brain death can now be determined, are the traditional criteria generally used to define death— the cessation of circulatory and respiratory functions within the body— outmoded and irrelevant?

219

Questions such as these and others are now so commonplace that they frequently occupy the headlines in our daily newspapers and often constitute the lead essays and articles in our most thoughtful magazines and journals. Moreover, increasing numbers of medical professionals, patients, and their families stand dazed and overwhelmed in physicians' offices, medical clinics, and hospitals throughout our country agonizingly confronting and desperately seeking just solutions to the life and death choices that lie before them. Faced with the often harrowing nature of this reality, many turn to religious tradition for direction and guidance. They ask the ethical authorities of their tradition to put forth principles that will guide judgments and to articulate reasons that will provide warrants for legitimating action.

Of course, making such determinations on the basis of a specific tradition is seldom a simple or an easy task. Modern literary criticism and theories of hermeneutics make clear that the reading of a religious tradition involves a nuanced and multilayered process. History teaches that values and principles evolve over time and indicates how deeply embedded such ideals and rules are in cultural and temporal contexts. Most significantly, anthropology reveals that a tradition's view of the nature of humanity and of humanity's relationship with God significantly informs the interpretive process. It is with these cautions and caveats in mind that I go on now to describe and analyze the dominant ways that Jewish ethicists have approached the sources and have characterized the ethos and traditions of Judaism in hope of guidance and direction on these mortal matters. Through an exploration and description of the major ways in which Jewish ethicists have in fact read the Jewish tradition to arrive at decisions on these questions, the essay is meant to highlight the critical role that methodology plays in rendering such judgments. It will argue that the different ways Jews approach their religious heritage is of significance in determining how Jewish medical ethics are to be done or, to put it in other terms, in determining what medical ethics are. These methodologies not only define who is competent to make such decisions, but, in doing so, show themselves possessed of profound implications for the normative judgment that might be rendered in a specific case.

Jewish medical ethics have been predominantly characterized by a methodology that one commentator has labeled "halakhic formalism." This classical mode of doing Jewish ethics seeks to identify precedents from the rich literature of rabbinic Judaism in order to extrapolate principles and norms that would yield authentic Jewish prescriptions on specific issues. Such an approach is hardly startling. After all, Judaism has preeminently grounded its authority in law and in the rabbinic interpretation of that law throughout its postbiblical history.[1] For over a millennium rabbis have employed responsa to apply the ideas and guides derived from the sacred texts of Judaism to the problems of a contemporary situation. Viewed in this way, Jewish medical ethics evidence the same methodological concerns and qualities that one would discover in any legal process.

This process, as David A. J. Richards has observed, displays two major characteristics. The first is that the judge, or the rabbi in our case, "infers the legal standards applicable to a particular situation from a body of so-called primary authority."[2] In Jewish law, this "body of so-called primary authority" includes both the Bible and the Talmud, which assumes a "statutory" role in the Jewish legal system, and an ongoing process of judicial opinions contained in responsa and codes that function in a "precedential" way. Here the interpretation of the law offered in the previous case (its holding) is seen to have a bearing on the adjudication of a contemporary case that deals, in the rabbi's opinion, with the same issue of law. A second feature of legal reasoning, related to but not identical with the first, is that of "reasoning by analogy." Rabbis, in this instance, not only take prior holdings on a comparable issue into account when rendering their decisions, but extend "principles of law found applicable to one set of fact patterns . . . to other fact patterns which are in relevant respects similar."[3]

Such an approach seems and, in many senses, is relatively straightforward. One simply plumbs the depths of Jewish law and discovers there the resources to resolve a perplexing moral issue. However, noting the method employed in such a moral exploration should not obscure the fact that genuine differences of opinion arise among diverse authorities as to the prescriptions the law yields on virtually every specific topic. Adherence to a common methodology does not preclude pluralism within the system. Authorities within any system of law can read precedents either stringently or leniently. They can assert that one set of precedents or values contained in the canon of a tradition is relevant to the matter at hand, while another group may assert that such precedents either have no bearing or have been completely misread. Affirmation of a common methodology in no way ensures a single substantive outcome.

An illustration of these points can easily be seen through an examination of several articles written by leading exemplars of "halakhic formalism" on the issue of the Jewish definition of death. Debate on this issue centers around whether Judaism considers what modern medicine terms "brain death" to be a sufficient criterion for establishing an individual as dead. All these writings cite an important talmudic text in tractate Yoma 85a as the *locus classicus* for the Jewish definition of death. Here the absence or cessation of breathing is regarded as the critical determinant of death. This definition is reinforced by passages in Maimonides' great code, the *Mishneh Torah*, Hilkhot Shabbat 2:19, and the subsequent, authoritative code of Joseph Karo, the *Shulḥan Arukh, Oraḥ Ḥayyim* 329:4. Furthermore, some later rabbinic authorities such as the Ḥatam Sofer, Rabbi Moses Schreiber of nineteenth-century Hungary, and Rabbi Eliezer Yehuda Waldenberg (Tzitz Eliezer) of twentieth-century Jerusalem, comment on this ruling in the Talmud and codes and expand the talmudic definition of death to include the cessation of cardiac activity. Thus, the classical rabbinic understanding of death, based as it is on the statutory and precedential sources of the Jewish legal tradition, involves the cessation of both cardiac and respiratory activities in the individual. Only then, when resuscitation is impossible, is the person considered deceased.

Virtually every single position advanced by leading traditionalist rabbis and doctors on the subject of the Jewish definition of death cites these passages and others in offering views of the Jewish definition of death. In so doing, the authors, in the words of Rabbi Herschel Schachter of Yeshiva University in New York, are doing what Jewish legal decisors (*poskim*) have done for centuries. They are juxtaposing "the particulars of [their] own case and various halakhic precedents and principles, thereby decid[ing] into which category [their] own case falls. Then [they] must apply these precedents and principles to the situation at hand."[4]

The problem in the case at hand, in Rabbi Schachter's opinion, is that "the situation of a brain-dead individual is unique to our generation."[5] Only in our day has medical technology been so advanced that brain death—the determination that there is no connection between the brain and the circulation of blood in the rest of the body—could be ascertained. How does such a development affect the rabbinic understanding and application of traditional Jewish sources on the issue of the definition of death? Can principles be extrapolated from them that will allow contemporary authorities to state whether brain death in fact constitutes death? The answers, as we shall see, are varied.

Rabbi J. David Bleich rules that, even if there is brain death and irreversible coma, these are not sufficient to establish a person as dead in Jewish law. Jewish sources on the subject, in Rabbi Bleich's opinion, clearly define death as the complete cessation of cardiac and respiratory activities with no hope for resuscitation. No advance in modern medical technology can alter these criteria as the decisive ones in offering a Jewish definition of death. Rabbi Bleich obviously reads and applies the sources of traditional Judaism quite literally on this matter.[6]

Dr. Fred Rosner and Rabbi Dr. Moshe David Tendler understand the issue somewhat differently. Although they cite the same classical sources that Rabbi Bleich does in approaching this question, they also employ a responsum by the late Rabbi Moshe Feinstein, perhaps the foremost Orthodox halakhic authority in twentieth-century America, as a warrant for their contention that "Jewish writings provide considerable evidence for the thesis that the brain and the brain stem control all bodily functions, including respiration and cardiac activity. It, therefore, follows that if there is irreversible and total cessation of all brain function, including that of the brain stem, the person is dead, even though there may still be some transient spontaneous cardiac activity."[7]

Dr. Rosner and Rabbi Tendler, in disagreeing with Rabbi Bleich, do not, in a certain sense, dispute his reading of the sources. Rather, they question whether the Yoma passage on which Rabbi Bleich and others in part construct their definition of death is relevant to the matter at hand. The Yoma passage, in their opinion, focuses on the absence of breathing and movement as a confirmation that death has occurred. It looks to the cessation of respiratory activity as a sign that death has taken place. In light of contemporary medical advances that allow an intensive care unit patient's every function to be monitored, more sophisticated standards for determining whether these activities have ceased can be established. However, even when such cessation has been established by the finest and most accurate tests medical science has to offer, they still do not provide a definition of death. They confirm only that death has occurred. In other words, Dr. Rosner and Rabbi Tendler assert, against Rabbi Bleich, that the Yoma passage is in effect irrelevant for providing criteria for establishing a Jewish definition of death. My interest here is not to judge whose reading of the source is correct. Instead it is to point out that even when authorities employ the same methodology, they may read the sources of a tradition in quite dissimilar ways.[8]

What, then, are the criteria that Rabbi Tendler and Dr. Rosner utilize to establish a Jewish definition of death? An understanding of how they do this will be crucial in illuminating the nature of how "halakhic formalists" go about the business of Jewish medical ethics and will reveal the pluralism inherent in this approach. Returning to Rabbi Feinstein's responsum, they report his contention that, if it can be medically determined that there is no circulation to the brain, the patient is equivalent to a decapitated person whose heart may still momentarily be beating. Such a person, according to Jewish law, is dead.[9] In other words, not all organs need cease functioning for death to be said to occur. "Physiologic decapitation," to quote Rabbi Tendler, "is sufficient to provide a definition of death." In our day, according to Dr. Rosner and Rabbi Tendler, such "physiologic decapitation" can be determined through testing for brain death.

Dr. Rosner and Rabbi Tendler, on the basis of the talmudic principle *shinnui ha-ittim,* "a changed reality," are able, in effect, to assert that talmudic texts must be read in accord with the judicial principle of "purposive interpretation." Scientific evidence and advances possess the right to guide and inform Jewish legal interpretation. In an era when sophisticated medical tests that could measure brain death were not available, Jewish law naturally employed the criteria of its day—the observation that breathing had ceased and that all external bodily movement had completely stopped—to confirm that death had occurred. However, in our day, when medical tests do exist that can determine that all brain-related functions have completely ceased, it is possible to contend that the classical definition of "respiratory and circulatory death" as constituting the crucial criteria in determining an individual's death must be understood in a broader way. "The classic 'respiratory and circulatory death' is," write Dr. Rosner and Rabbi Tendler, "in reality brain death."[10]

Other authorities, notably Rabbi Aharon Soloveichik, sharply disagree with Dr. Rosner and Rabbi Tendler on this, just as the latter dissented from Rabbi Bleich.[11] Once more, the point here is not to suggest what a normative reading of Jewish law on this topic might be. Instead, in the context of our discussion, it is apparent that this approach to Jewish medical ethics, while text centered, is hardly univocal. Different authorities read the same texts in diverse ways. They offer different opinions as to which texts provide appropriate analogs for understanding a contemporary situation. Rabbi Tendler and Dr. Rosner believe that the concept of "physiologic decapitation" is germane to this discussion and warranted by a reading of the sources. Rabbi Soloveichik sharply disagrees. Rabbi Bleich asserts that the traditional halakhic criteria for defining death must be narrowly and literally understood. Dr. Rosner and Rabbi Tendler contend that such texts must be comprehended in light of their "true intent," and that this intent is best captured in view of contemporary medical advances. A common methodological approach should not obscure the fact that the interpretive process is nuanced and variegated. Although the methodology of "halakhic formalism" may be text centered, the judgments that emerge from such an approach are often multivalent.

"Halakhic formalism" is characterized by more than its attention to classical texts. It is also transdenominational, that is, not only Orthodox authorities have adopted this methodology in approaching the complex issues of medical ethics. It has also been the predominant manner in which non-Orthodox rabbis have attempted to deal with questions in this area. A glance at Jewish writings on the issue of euthanasia is illustrative of this. Addressing the question of whether a terminally ill patient suffering from excruciating pain can request a medicine that will simultaneously relieve his agony and hasten his death, Rabbi Solomon Freehof, the leading Reform rabbinical author of modern responsa, responds that "for a man to ask that his life be ended sooner is the equivalent of his committing suicide. Suicide is definitely forbidden by Jewish law."[12] Rabbi Elliot Dorff, a leading conservative theologian and ethicist, writes on the same issue in an identical way. As Dorff phrases it, "Judaism prohibits murder in all circumstances, and it views all forms of active euthanasia as the equivalent of murder. That is true even if the patient asks to be killed."[13]

Orthodox Rabbi Immanuel Jakobovits also arrives at the same conclusion. Chief Rabbi of Great Britain and author of the definitive *Jewish Medical Ethics*, Jakobovits observes, "There is no question . . . to Judaism, of absolute and unconditional opposition to any form of direct or active euthanasia. . . . Any physician deliberately causing a patient to die, under whatever conditions of debility or suffering, is regarded as committing an act of first degree murder. Nor would any account whatsoever be taken of the wishes of the patient. We are no more masters of our own lives than we are masters of anyone else's. . . . We have no right . . . to forego our absolute claim to life by giving consent to its destruction."[14] Finally, Rabbi Bleich, already cited above, concurs with these sentiments and issues the following opinion:

> Elimination of pain is certainly a legitimate and laudable goal. According to some authorities it is encompassed within the general obligation to heal. . . . Yet when the dual goals of avoidance of pain and preservation of life come into conflict with one another, Judaism recognizes the paramount value and sanctity of life and, accordingly, assigns priority to preservation of life. Thus, a number of authorities have expressly stated that non-treatment or withdrawal of treatment in order for the patient to be freed from pain by death constitutes euthanasia and is not countenanced by Judaism. This remains the case even if the patient himself pleads to be permitted to die.[15]

The issue for us here is not whether the tradition could or should have been construed by these authorities in a different manner. As Rabbi Bleich has observed, and as Rabbi Jakobovits and others have noted, the commandment to relieve the pain of a suffering patient is mandated by Jewish law. Rabbi Freehof, in fact, expands on a view of this mandate and, in the end, issues a lenient ruling on this matter. He submits, on the basis of talmudic passages in Avodah Zarah 27a and b and Ketubot 104a, that "we may take definite action to relieve pain, even if it is of some risk to the last hours. . . . It is possible to reason as follows: It is true that the medicine to relieve the pain may weaken his heart, but does not the great pain itself weaken his heart? May it not be that relieving the pain may strengthen him more than the medicine might weaken him? At all events, it is a matter of judgment."[16] Rabbi Freehof, informed by the commandment to relieve suffering, offers the possibility that the fulfillment of this mandate does not abrogate the traditional directive to lengthen life in this instance. In so doing, he obviously departs from the ruling put forth by other halakhic authorities on this question. Furthermore, in his view of the revelatory character of Jewish law, he and Rabbi Dorff, too, will undoubtedly differ from the Orthodox rabbis cited here. However, once Freehof employs the same methodology that they do and elects to ground his judgments in the statutes and precedent of the Jewish legal tradition, any difference between him and them is incidental to the methodology he employs. In theory, other authorities could rule as he did.

Freehof's reading of the texts of the rabbinic tradition here is certainly informed by extralegal considerations such as personality and disposition. These cause him to apply precedents from the tradition that the others do not affirm. However, this has nothing to do with the methodology that is employed. His manner of making a decision is identical to the others. The pluralism evidenced here has nothing to do with Jewish denominationalism. It is qualitatively, from a methodological standpoint, no different than the difference of opinion we saw above between Rabbi Bleich and Rabbi Tendler on the matter of a Jewish definition of death. Furthermore, while Rabbi Freehof's own inclinations may have caused him to read the sources and cite the precedents for his decision in the manner that he did, this in no way distinguishes him methodologically from Orthodox halakhists who also admit extralegal considerations as factors that influence their own reading of the tradition. For example, Rabbi Faitel Levin of Melbourne, Australia, another prominent Orthodox authority in this area, cites the degradation of human life evidenced in the Holocaust as a factor, albeit not the decisive one, in his contention that Jewish law cannot countenance active euthanasia in any form, even to alleviate the suffering of a dying patient. Such a policy, he feels, would relativize the value of life.[17] In short, the methodological direction provided by "halakhic formalism" does not preclude lenient or demand stringent decisions. Tremendous discretion in how the sources are read remains with the rabbi who is issuing the decision. Rather, the methodology simply demands that the decision be warranted by a text taken from the tradition. The writings of Freehof, Dorff, and all the Orthodox authorities discussed here reveal the same text centeredness, the same methodological grounding of their decisions in warrants derived from the literary canon of Judaism.

One final point about the nature of "halakhic formalism" must be made if a full appreciation of the character of this methodology is to result. Simply put, individual autonomy is not prized as an independent variable in this approach to Jewish medical ethics. Great concern for the individual is clearly present here. The suffering of persons and the nature of their lives are often taken into compassionate account. However, judgments are ultimately made, as Rabbi Jakobovits phrases it, by "competent moral authorities—rabbis in the case of those who submit to Jewish law."[18] Rabbis might decide, in a given case, that the law can be interpreted in such a way as to provide a coherent exception to the rule that Jewish law prohibits active euthanasia. This, as we saw, is precisely what Rabbi Freehof did. Nevertheless, the decision must ultimately be made, according to Rabbi Bleich, not by the patient nor by his or her family, but by "a qualified rabbinic authority for adjudication on a case-by-case basis."[19] This is because, as Conservative Rabbi Joel Roth, Professor of Talmud at the Jewish Theological Seminary of America, observes in a strong, but accurate, description of this position, the "meaning of the Torah," the source for competent Jewish ethical judgment on these matters, is in the hands of the rabbis. "Rabbinic authority," Roth writes, "is, in theory, unbounded. . . . Rabbinic interpretation of the law is, as it were, the never-ending revelation of the will of God."[20]

The writings of every authority cited on the issue of active euthanasia reveal a refusal to recognize the ultimate right of individuals to make autonomous decisions concerning the nature of the treatment they will receive. Even when a terminally ill patient suffering unbearable agony requests that his or her life be ended or be permitted to expire, it is the rabbi, informed by considerations for the patient and by competent medical advice, who makes, in theory, the final decision. Such matters, from the standpoint of "halakhic formalism," are not left to individuals, their families, or physicians, but to rabbinic authority. "Halakhic formalism," precisely because it is textually centered, can grant supreme authority only to those who have studied and mastered the texts—the rabbis. Again, this does not preclude a pluralism of views. It does not mean that decisions cannot be kindly and merciful. It does indicate that individual autonomy is not a paramount, not perhaps even a secondary, value in the system.

A trend toward developing an alternative approach to the dominant one of "halakhic formalism" has begun to emerge in recent years. The reasons for this have been suggested in an insightful article written recently by Rabbi Daniel Gordis, a member of the faculty at the (Conservative) University of Judaism in Los Angeles. In an article entitled "Wanted—The Ethical in Jewish Bio-Ethics," Rabbi Gordis suggests that developments in medical technology have been so dazzling in recent years that a precedent-based classical approach to issues of Jewish bio-ethics is simply inadequate to address contemporary realities. Gordis, for example, points to the fact that A.I.D. has been labeled adultery by many Jewish ethicists if the donor's semen is other than the husband's. "In an age in which adultery is a serious societal issue," writes Rabbi Gordis, "employing *it* as the precedent for A.I.D. both minimizes the moral claim against 'real' adultery, and lessens the seriousness with which objective observers will view legitimate claims that *halakhah* has potential relevance in other realms."[21]

Gordis goes on to provide examples of what he considers unwarranted extrapolation of principles and norms from Jewish halakhic and aggadic writings on other modern medical moral dilemmas. Although his contentions about the relevance of precedents drawn from the sources of Judaism to modern medical ethics may be somewhat exaggerated, the significant point is that this belief leads Gordis to assert that "halakhic formalism" provides an inadequate methodology for doing Jewish medical ethics. It is wrong or, at best, foolish to search the precedents of the Jewish tradition in such a narrow, case-law fashion to find answers to matters of contemporary bioethics. Instead he turns to what can be identified as theological anthropology for a solution to his methodological dilemma; that is, Rabbi Gordis states that the texts of Judaism must be examined to see what they have to say about the nature of what it means to be human. Furthermore, in seeking an answer to such a question, the ancillary issue of humanity's relationship with God arises. If one were to receive answers to these broader questions, then it might well be that Jewish medical ethics would draw normative conclusions in a far different way than it does with a methodology based on precedent.[22]

Such a methodology, though nascent and somewhat inchoate—reminding one at times of a theory of moral intuitionism—already has its champions. The maverick Orthodox Rabbi Irving Greenberg, one of the most prominent interpreters of Jewish tradition in North America, labels such a methodological approach "covenantal." This "covenantal" approach to Jewish medical ethics, like its precedent-oriented counterpart of "halakhic formalism," is transdenominational. Representatives from both the Orthodox and liberal Jewish communities have championed this mode of doing Jewish ethics. Among its most prominent representatives have been Rabbi David Hartman of Jerusalem and Rabbi Eugene Borowitz of the Hebrew Union College-Jewish Institute of Religion in New York. This approach is marked by the dialectical, personal model of relationship between God and humanity found in the Bible. It affirms the belief that "humankind is created so as to be God's partner in completing creation."[23] This means that God's covenant with Israel does not restrict human freedom, but presupposes it. As Rabbi Borowitz avers, "Though God's sovereign rule of the universe is utterly unimpeachable, people under the covenant need not surrender their selfhood to God. If anything, to participate properly in the alliance they must affirm their freedom, for they are called to acceptance and resolve, not servility."[24] Or, as Rabbi Hartman phrases it, "The freedom of the beloved [humanity] precludes the possibility of absolute control [by God] and self-sufficiency [by persons]."[25] A covenantal mode of doing Jewish ethics calls for a balance between the belief in and reliance on God on the one hand and the affirmation of human autonomy on the other.

An authentic Jewish moral theory, from this covenantal perspective, must neglect neither God nor persons. "For Jewish ethics," as Rabbi Michael Morgan, Professor of Philosophy at Indiana University, has stated, "is by its very nature rooted in a Divine Command that is imposed and yet freely accepted."[26] Jewish medical ethics must involve a dialectic in which both God and humanity play an active role. This means that one must search out the tradition for those precedents relevant to the making of an ethical decision. Not to do so would provide an unwarranted break with a huge dimension of the tradition and would deny Jews the continuity and wisdom such precedents have to offer. However, this theory also affirms that since human beings are created in the image of God, then they share in God's power. Human life and human wisdom, seen from this perspective, are reflections of the power of God. Such an approach, as the covenantal ethicists perceive it, does not usurp the power of God. Rather, it reflects the innate dignity inherent in both God and God's creation. In short, human autonomy—the ability of individual persons to make and to act on their own ethical decisions—derives from the freedom that God has given persons.[27] The affirmation of human autonomy seen in this dialectic is not the product of enlightenment thought. Rather, it receives a divine, religious warrant.

The implications of this methodology for Jewish decision making in the area of bioethics can be seen in an article entitled "Toward a Covenantal Ethic of Medicine," written by Rabbi Greenberg. In this paper, Rabbi Greenberg argues that the dialectical interplay between "power and partnership" that is the mark of the relationship between God and humanity in the Bible provides the proper model for Jewish medical ethics as well. This means, in part, that people are empowered to become more and more like God. They are charged by God with responsibility for their lives and are given permission to seek mastery and control over their environment. If someone asks, "What are the limits?" Rabbi Greenberg contends the covenantal response "is that the limit is nonexistent."[28]

Interestingly, Rabbi Greenberg, like Rabbi Levin above, cites the Holocaust in support of his position. However, instead of drawing the lesson from it that the Holocaust simply cheapened the value of human life,

Greenberg states that the proper lesson to be derived from this horrific event is that bureaucracy, when left unchecked, can totally deprive people of power and lead to excesses of evil behavior. The Holocaust demonstrates what can occur when an "ethic of powerlessness" dominates. Greenberg desires to assert an ethic of power, an ethic of human beings charged with responsibility and control for their own decisions, as the proper Jewish model to be employed in our time. Autonomy within the covenantal dialectic, so understood, would mean not only that people frame actions and rules for their own lives in concert with the tradition, it also involves an affirmation of the person's right to act upon that determination. The covenantal model is one of partnership in which human beings have the legitimate right to exercise a high degree of control over their own lives.

This means that individuals have the right to ask quality of life, not only quantity of life questions. Greenberg states:

> The original birth control prohibition in Jewish law reflects the fear that human control over who shall be created, who shall be given life, is somehow robbing God of his power. What is really involved . . . is an ethical trade-off: the quality of life versus the quantity of life. It is necessary to know that quantity is important. It is also essential to know that quality matters. If the marriage needs more time, if the mother . . . cannot handle the number of children, then it is ethical *not* to have the child rather than have it. This is the balancing act that has to be undertaken.[29]

It is clear that this covenantal approach to Jewish medical ethics possesses implications that radically distinguish it from the precedent-oriented approach of the "halakhic formalists." If we look at the issue of active euthanasia posed above, the covenantal ethicist, following Greenberg's methodology, might well reach a different conclusion than the classical Jewish ethicist concerning the decision to terminate life. Quality of life concerns could certainly enter the picture.

Far more significantly, it is impossible to imagine that the rabbi would be designated by the "covenantal ethicist" as the ultimate arbiter of what was moral in a case such as this. The rabbi could certainly occupy a legitimate role as a consultant and could provide the patient, the family, and the physician with information drawn from the precedents of Jewish tradition on this matter. The patient, in the end, might well choose to follow them. However, and this is the crucial point, it is the patient who would be empowered to make this decision—not the doctor, not the rabbi, not his or her family. The person's autonomy as a covenantal creature standing in relationship with God would ultimately be affirmed as the highest value in the system. All this is not to maintain that an individual is necessarily any better equipped to make an ethical decision than an institution or an outsider. It is also not to assert that a decision to terminate the life of a hopelessly ill patient suffering horrible pain is necessarily a more worthy moral choice than another one. For purposes of this paper, the substantive decision that might be made is beside the point. What is critical is that human autonomy, seen from this methodological perspective, is one pole on which Jewish medical ethics rests. Although a great deal of more rigorous work on the nature of this approach must be done, the direction already charted by its advocates clearly distinguishes it from the approach of the "halakhic formalists" and has far-reaching implications for the normative conclusions that Jewish medical ethics might ultimately draw.

The questions posed to humanity today by advances in medical science are truly frightening. There are no easy answers. Moreover, even when persons affirm a common approach to a religious tradition, the conclusions for normative practice can be many. However, I hope that this presentation has sensitized us not only to the way in which Jewish medical ethics have been done in our day, but to the important role that methodology occupies in the way that rabbis and individual Jews read their tradition for ethical guidance on the mortal issues. We Jews like to think of ourselves as *rahmanim b'nei rahmanim,* merciful people who are the children of merciful people. May our reading of our tradition on these mortal matters be, in view of these methodologies, a fulfillment of this vision as we deal with the realities of human suffering and human healing in our lives.

ACKNOWLEDGMENTS

I would like to express my gratitude to Lee Bycel, Michael Signer, and Stanley Chyet for having discussed issues in this paper with me. I would especially like to thank my colleague William Cutter, who gave me extensive bibliographical assistance and who provoked me to think about many of the issues discussed in this presentation.

NOTES AND REFERENCES

1.   Daniel H. Gordis, "Wanted—The Ethical in Jewish Bioethics," *Judaism* 38 (1989): 29.

2.   David A. J. Richards, *The Moral Criticism of the Law* (Encino and Belmont, CA: Dickenson Publishing Co., 1977), 26.

3.   *Ibid.,* 28.

4. Herschel Schachter, "Determining the Time of Death," *The Journal of Halacha and Contemporary Society,* 17 (1989): 32.

5. *Ibid.*

6. J. David Bleich, *Contemporary Halakhic Problems* (New York: KTAV, 1977), 372–393.

7. Fred Rosner and Moshe David Tendler, "Determining the Time of Death," *The Journal of Halacha and Contemporary Society* 17 (1989): 17.

8. *Ibid.,* 24.

9. *Ibid.*

10. *Ibid.,* 27.

11. Aharon Soloveichik, "Determining the Time of Death," *The Journal of Halacha and Contemporary Society* 17 (1989): 41–48.

12. Walter Jacob, ed. *American Reform Responsa* (New York: Central Conference of American Rabbis, 1983), 254.

13. Elliot N. Dorff, "Choose Life: A Jewish Perspective on Medical Ethics," "University Papers, 4, 1 (Los Angeles: University of Judaism, 1985), 17.

14. Immanuel Jakobovits, "Ethical Problems Regarding the Termination of Life," in *Jewish Values in Bioethics,* Levi Meier, ed. (New York: Human Sciences Press, 1986), 90.

15. J. David Bleich, *Judaism and Healing: Halakhic Perspectives* (New York: KTAV, 1981), 137.

16. Jacob, *op. cit.,* 256–257.

17. Faitel Levin, *Halacha, Medical Science, and Technology: Perspectives on Contemporary Halacha Issues* (New York and Jerusalem: Maznaim Publishing Corporation, 1987), 64–65.

18. Jakobovits, *op. cit.,* 91.

19. Bleich, *Judaism and Healing,* 144.

20. Joel Roth, *The Halakhic Process* (New York: KTAV, 1987), 133.

21. Gordis, *op. cit.,* 29.

22. *Ibid.,* 28–40.

23. Irving Greenberg, "Toward a Covenantal Ethic of Medicine," in *Jewish Values in Bioethics,* Levi Meier, ed. (New York: Human Sciences Press, 1986), 124–149.

24. Eugene B. Borowitz, *Choices in Modern Jewish Thought* (New York: Behrman House, 1983), 367–368.

25. David Hartman, "Moral Uncertainties in the Practice of Medicine," *The Journal of Medicine and Philosophy* 4 (1979): 100.

26. Michael Morgan, "Jewish Ethics after the Holocaust," *The Journal of Religious Ethics* 12 (1984): 259.

27. Eugene B. Borowitz, "The Autonomous Self and the Commanding Community," *Theological Studies* 45 (1984): 48–49.

28. Greenberg, *op. cit.,* 137.

29. *Ibid.,* 145.

14

How to Draw Guidance from a Heritage: A Catholic Approach to Mortal Choices

Richard A. McCormick, S.J.

Our theme asks how we should draw guidance from our religious heritage when we are faced with making mortal choices. I will address that issue from the perspective of the Catholic heritage. What does this heritage have to say to "mortal choices"?

Let me say by way of introduction that the term "guidance" is well chosen and should be emphasized. It is not the same as "solution," "answer," or "conclusion." The sources of faith in Catholic tradition are to enlighten conscience, not replace it. I point this out because of the reemergence in our time of a certain Catholic magisteriolatry in which principle and application, substance and formulation get collapsed into indistinctness in a misguided total reliance on authority.

Let me divide my considerations into two parts: theological framework and practical application.

THEOLOGICAL FRAMEWORK

Some grow very nervous at the mention of theology or a "religious approach" to mortal choices. Undoubtedly some entertain very subjectivistic notions of religion and regard it as an intrusion into an autonomous science and art. Some imagine a theologian citing a text from scripture as decisive for clinical practice as in televangelical practice. Worse yet some conjure up a pope or bishop, supposedly in prior possession of arcane wisdom that yields solutions to difficult dilemmas. Even though some theologians may be biblical fundamentalists and eth-

ical threats, and even though not all hierarchical processes are rehabilitated to contemporary times, these fears are overall unfounded and
represent distortions of and departures from the Catholic heritage.

That heritage is anchored in faith in the meaning and decisive significance of God's covenant with human beings, especially as manifested in
the saving incarnation of Jesus Christ and the revelation of His final
coming, His eschatological kingdom that is now aborning but will finally
only be given. Faith in these events and loyalty to their central figure
yield a decisive way of viewing and intending the world, of interpreting
its meaning and hierarchizing its values. Rather than a thesaurus of
answers, the sources of faith function as narratives. From narratives or a
story come perspectives, themes, and insights, not always or chiefly
concrete action guides.

To see what these perspectives, themes, insights—as related to medical ethics and its mortal choices—might be, let us attempt to disengage
some key elements of the Christian story, and from a Catholic reading
and living of it. One might not be too far off with the following:

1. God is the author and preserver of life. We are "made in His
    image."
2. Thus life is a gift, a trust. It has great worth because of the value
    He is placing in it (Thielicke's "alien dignity").
3. God places great value in it because He is also (besides being
    author) the end, purpose of life.
4. We are on a pilgrimage, having here no lasting home.
5. God has dealt with us in many ways. But His supreme epiphany
    of Himself (and our potential selves) is His Son Jesus Christ.
6. In Jesus' life, death, and resurrection we have been totally trans-
    formed into "new creatures," into a community of the trans-
    formed. Sin and death have met their victor.
7. The ultimate significance of our lives consists in developing this
    new life.
8. The spirit is given to us to guide and inspire us on this journey.
9. The ultimate destiny of our combined journeys is the "coming of
    the Kingdom," and the return of the glorified Christ to claim the
    redeemed world.
10. Thus we are offered in and through Jesus Christ eternal life. Just
    as Jesus has overcome death (and now lives), so will we who
    cling to Him, place our faith and hope in Him, and take Him as
    our law and model.
11. This good news, this covenant with us has been entrusted to a
    people, a people to be nourished and instructed by shepherds.
12. These people should continuously remember and thereby make

present Christ in His death and resurrection at the Eucharistic meal.

13. The chief and central manifestation of this new life in Christ is love for each other (not a flaccid "niceness," but a love that shapes itself in concrete forms of justice, gratitude, forbearance, chastity, etc.).

If we are thinking *theologically* (obviously I refer to Christian theology) about the ethical problems of biomedicine, it is out of such framework, context, or story that we will think. The very meaning, purpose, and value of a person is grounded and ultimately explained in this story. Since that is the case, the story itself is the overarching foundation and criterion of morality. It stands in judgment of all human meaning and actions. Actions that are incompatible with this story are thereby *morally wrong*. In its *Declaration on Euthanasia*, the Sacred Congregation for the Doctrine of the Faith made reference to "Christ, who through His life, death, and resurrection, has given a *new meaning to existence*."[1] If that is true (and Christians believe it is), then to neglect that meaning is to neglect the most important thing about ourselves, to cut ourselves off from the fullness of our own reality.

The Christian story tells us the ultimate meaning of ourselves and the world. In doing so, it tells us the kind of people we ought to be, the goods we ought to pursue, the dangers we ought to avoid, and the kind of world we ought to seek. It provides the backdrop or framework that ought to shape our individual decisions. When decision making is separated from this framework, it loses its perspective. It can easily become a merely rationalistic and sterile ethic subject to the distortions of self-interested perspectives and cultural drifts, a kind of contracted etiquette with no relation to the ultimate meaning of persons. (Indeed, even when our deliberations are nourished by the biblical narrative, they do not escape the *reliquiae peccati* in us.)

A medical symbol of this separation is a statement of Terry Kennedy, a spokesman for Nassau Hospital, in the Brother Fox case. Kennedy stated: "Our mission is to do all that we can do to maintain life." The implication is that mere life (ventilation and circulation) has a human value as such and must be maintained. A similar statement was issued by the Missouri Supreme Court in the Nancy Cruzan case when it said the state's interest in life is "unqualified." I believe that even some Catholic theologians and bishops err when they refer to years of life in a persistent vegetative state as "a great benefit to the patient." The Christian story will not, in my judgment, support this. Once a value judgment is separated from the story that displays our meaning, it begins to be controlled by mere technology.

Here we happen on the inherent danger of medicine practiced in a western secularized society. In such a society (by definition), the story that reveals the meaning of life is no longer widely functional. Meaning must be derived from elsewhere, and decisions shaped in other ways. Thus in our secularized society we have (1) the assertion of autonomy as the controlling value of the person, and (2) the canonization of pluralism as instrumental to it. The modern liberal secularized society sees its task as protecting the individual's autonomy to do his/her own thing. The function of the state is to guarantee and protect the right of noninterference. I am not attacking autonomy. It is surely a precious value. But it is the condition of moral behavior, not its exhaustive definition. To view it as exhaustive is to ask the state to remain neutral on our most treasured and basic values (e.g., the family). In this context Daniel Callahan has noted that "general solutions and binding group norms need to be worked out that are of more than a consensual or procedural kind."[2] He continues: "If personal morality comes down to nothing more than the exercise of free choice, with no principles available for moral judgment of the quality of those choices, then we will have a 'moral vacuum.'"

It is precisely the secularism of western society that makes the humane use of our technology seem so problematic. We have distanced ourselves from the very matrix (story) that is the only complete indicator of the truly human. How can we be humane without full knowledge of the human? Considerations such as these lead to the assertion that theology is utterly essential to bioethical discussions. It does not give us concrete answers or ready-made rules. But it does tell us who we are, where we come from, where we are going, who we ought to be becoming. It is only against such understandings that our concrete deliberations can remain truly humane and promote our best interests.

Vatican II puts it as follows: "Faith throws a new light on everything, manifests God's design for man's total vocation, and thus directs the mind to solutions which are fully human."[3] It further stated: "But only God, who created man to His own image and ransoms him from sin, provides a fully adequate answer to these questions. This He does through what He has revealed in Christ His Son, who became man. Whoever follows after Christ, the perfect man, becomes himself more of a man."[4]

The Catholic tradition, in dealing with concrete moral problems, has encapsulated the way faith "directs the mind to solutions" in the phrase "reason informed by faith." Thus Pius XII, when speaking of the suppression of consciousness, stated that it was "permitted by natural morality and *in keeping with* the spirit of the Gospel."[5] The Congregation for the Doctrine of the Faith in the *Declaration on Euthanasia* referred to "human and Christian prudence." "Reason informed by faith" is neither reason replaced by faith, nor reason without faith. It is reason shaped by faith and, in my judgment, this shaping takes the form of perspectives, themes, insights associated with the story that aid us to construe the world.

PRACTICAL APPLICATION

What has the Christian story and theology offered to us as guidance where mortal choices are concerned? A *value judgment* and a *policy*.

Value Judgment

The fact that we are pilgrims, that Christ has overcome death and lives, that we will also live with Him, yields a general value judgment on the meaning and value of life as we now live it. It can be formulated as follows: life is a basic good but not an absolute one. It is basic because, as the Congregation for the Doctrine of Faith worded it, it is the "necessary source and condition of every human activity and of all society."[6] It is not absolute because there are higher goods for which life can be sacrificed (glory of God, salvation of souls, service of one's brethren, etc.). Thus in *John* (15:13): "There is no greater love than this: to lay down one's life for one's friends." Therefore laying down one's life for another cannot be contrary to the faith or story or meaning of humankind. It is, after Jesus' example, life's greatest fulfillment, even though it is the end of life as we now know it. Negatively, we could word this value judgment as follows: Death is an evil but not an absolute or unconditioned one.

Policy or Basic Attitude

This value judgment has immediate relevance for care of the ill and dying. It issues in a basic attitude or policy: Not all means must be used to preserve life. Why? Pius XII in a 1952 address to the International Congress of Anesthesiologists stated: "A more strict obligation would be too burdensome for most men and would render the attainment of the higher, more important good too difficult. Life, health, all temporal activities are in fact subordinated to spiritual ends."[7] In other words, there are higher values than life in the living of it. There are also higher values in the dying of it.

What Pius XII was saying, then, is that forcing (morally) one to take all means is tantamount to forcing attention and energies on a subordinate good in a way that prejudices a higher good, even eventually making it unrecognizable as a good. Excessive concern for the temporal is at some point neglect of the eternal. An obligation to use all means to preserve life would be a devaluation of human life, since it would remove life from the context or story that is the source of its ultimate value.

Thus the Catholic tradition has moved between two extremes: medicomoral optimism or vitalism (which preserves life with all means, at any cost no matter what its condition) and medicomoral pessimism (which actively kills when life becomes onerous, dysfunctional, boring). Merely technological judgments could easily fall into either of these two traps.

Thus far theology. It yields a value judgment and a general policy or attitude. It provides the framework for subsequent moral reasoning. It tells us that life is a gift with a purpose and destiny. Dying is the last or waning moments of this "new creature." At this point moral reasoning (reason informed by faith) must assume its proper responsibilities to answer the following questions: (1) What means ought to be used, what need not be? (2) What shall we call such means? (3) Who enjoys the prerogative and/or duty of decision making? (4) What is to be done with now incompetent and always incompetent patients in critical illness? The sources of faith do not, in my judgment, provide direct answers to these questions.

This is the way, I submit, that the Catholic heritage provides guidance. It does not make decisions. Rather it informs and nourishes the decision-maker. If we look for more or settle for less, we may well part company with the evidence.

But a final warning note needs to be sounded. I have referred to a value judgment and a policy. There is a close relationship. It is clear that the value judgment originates and supports the policy. What is not so clear—but ought to be—is that mistaken policy applications can loosen our grasp on the basic value judgment itself. Thus mistaken judgments about what it is appropriate to do with and for Nancy Cruzan in her persistent vegetative state can separate us from the substance of Catholic tradition, a thing I think has happened in some recent analyses.

NOTES AND REFERENCES

1.   *Declaration on Euthanasia* (Vatican City: Vatican Polyglot Press, 1980). Also in *Origins* 10 (1980): 154–157.

2.   Daniel Callahan, "Shattuck Lecture: Contemporary Biomedical Ethics," *New England Journal of Medicine* 302, 22 (1980): 1232.

3.   *The Documents of Vatican II* (New York: America Press, 1966), 209.

4. *Ibid.*, 240.

5. *The Pope Speaks* 4 (1957): 45; AAS [*Acta Apostolicae Sedis*—Ed.] 48 (1957): 129–147.

6. Cf. note 1.

7. AAS [*Acta Apostolicae Sedis*—Ed.] 49 (1957): 1031–1032.

15

How to Draw Guidance from a Heritage: A Protestant Approach to Mortal Choices

Martin E. Marty

RELIGIOUS HERITAGES AND THE LARGER CULTURE

All religions are "about" being born and dying. Most of them have interest in the moral life and ethics. Western faiths and others that have linear views of history are preoccupied with time.[1] Modern religions accent choice. We need guidance when approaching mortal choices. Religions come to us as traditions, as heritages.[2] Virtually every word in my assigned title suggests reasons why people of faith and custodians of faith traditions have much at stake when people face mortal choices.

The world in which people pursue health and practice medicine today is not arranged to make it easy for the society at large or even for subcultures to draw guidance from these heritages. As a secular society, it is officially and often in practice constituted so that it does not or cannot listen to the words of faith communities.[3] As a pluralist society, it is officially committed to giving no more notice to a religious voice than a nonreligious one, to favoring one religion over another; yet it must also not put up barriers against the use of the language of faith in debate over choice.[4] As a liberal society, it moves more by skeptical rationality than by religious reasoning; in practice it treats religious differences with tolerance bordering on indifference and pays little respect to the "thickness" of faith communities; it relies on individualism and has difficulty responding to communities at all.[5] Yet people find a liberal society spiritually unsatisfying, and express themselves religiously within its bounds.

In this republic, to which for practical purposes I shall restrict my inquiry and comments, it is also impossible for religion and society *not* to interact. The people of particular faiths and the people of the general culture necessarily confront each other on important issues. For that matter, the same citizens make up much of the scientific, healing, and ethical communities, on one hand, and the religious communities, on the other. Further, passionately religious people want their faith reckoned with in public policy and private choice. Meanwhile scientific and political leadership indicates increasing openness to the religious heritages, sometimes out of a positive interest in discovery and sometimes out of a defensive interest in not offending or alienating constituencies.

Those three paragraphs are densely packed with propositions, and some of them need unpacking.

THE INTERESTS OF RELIGIOUS HERITAGES

In the first case, it is important to remember that most religions were born in no small part as healing cults and that most of the religions in our republic also have a strong interest in morals and ethics. Some faiths of the sort once called "primitive" and others called "Eastern" exist chiefly for the interpretation of an existing universe, for coming to terms with it. But the Abrahamaic, Jerusalemaic, biblical faiths—Judaism, Christianity, Islam—and the Enlightenment philosophy of religion influenced by Western biblicism, to say nothing of other religions that have been partly shaped by and in this environment, move beyond interpretation and coping. They demand obedience from followers and offer them guidance.

Thus adherents respond to calls: "Hear, O Israel," or "Thou shalt love," or "Submit," the first and key words in three heritages. The calls are spoken in a context of urgency, for history is seen as moving, and people live lives of destiny in a universe marked also by finitude, contingency, and transience. So time is freighted with meaning. There are special times: the day of the Lord, a *kairos,* a moment of summing up decision. The concept of choosing is old within these traditions: One may be called to conversion by them, or to "turning" and becoming faithful to a covenant within them. But modernity invests choice with special urgency. Peter Berger has characterized modern life as containing a "heretical imperative," recalling that the ancient word *haeresis,* which stands behind the word "heresy," meant "choice."[6] To be modern is, in part, to have moved from repose within a single tradition to an awareness of the intermingling of traditions, the lure of many heritages, the freedom to pick and choose elements among them.

Almost in passing, I mentioned that religions come to us as heritages, as traditions. Even millennial and utopian religions, eager as they are to see the birth of a wholly new universe and epoch, draw all their words, images, metaphors, and promises from past experience. American philosophers such as William James may define religion in connection with the instantaneous,[7] and the Marxist philosopher Ernst Bloch liked to stress the "infatuation with the possible," the interest in the *novum*, the new, within biblical faith,[8] yet expressions of faith through time get consolidated in stories, in corporate memories, in organizations and institutions, in schools that keep alive and nurture heritages.

As important as it is to stress the bearing of religious heritages on our topics, it is also important to concentrate on how hard it is to reach to them for guidance. Even new religious traditions such as Mormonism draw on canons shaped centuries before the modern scientific revolution or the invention of the republican polity. The religions tend to come as revelations, disclosures, or utterances from Yahweh, the "Abba" of Jesus Christ, or Allah; from unseen orders and from beyond horizons available to those who do not believe in them.[9] The texts address a world that did not anticipate the technology that has so greatly increased the world of choice. They often assume that all other traditions are wrong about choice and about the faith that lies behind it, and anticipate the life of religious communities that are either persecuted by dominant regimes or have a regime and a territory all to themselves.[10] Modern republics in their polity protect themselves against any of these faith communities or heritages gaining a monopoly or even hegemony.

DRAWING ON RELIGIOUS HERITAGES TODAY

The custodians of and respondents to these heritages today live in a world described as *Entzaubert*, "disenchanted," formally desacralized.[11] A modern legislature, university, laboratory, or clinic may be made up of people who are respectful of a religious heritage, but it cannot constitute itself on the faith assumptions that are inaccessible to most people who are members of its agencies. Judaism, Christianity, Islam, and so many other faith traditions speak to us across great divides created by the Renaissance, Enlightenment, and Modernity.[12] They are particular, and thus seem to be more difficult to approach than are would-be universalisms, such as Platonic and Aristotelian philosophy, which also antedate the rise of science and liberal democracy.

The news these years is, however, that scientists, academics, and republicans, often while expressing some understandable resistance or wariness and more often tardily and grudgingly, are coming to see that somehow they must recognize the people who draw guidance from these heritages and, thus, the heritages themselves. Indeed, in many cases late in secular, pluralist, and liberal histories, millions insist on drawing guidance more from these heritages than from philosophy itself, from academic expressions of ethics, or from patterns of decision based only on "secular rationality."[13] Even strategically and self-defensively they have to be aware of the religious commitments. Legislators know that, for instance, they can lose their political life if they are unaware of religious voices that are "pro-life" or that they have no choice but to listen to those who are "pro-choice." Lawmakers more positively take into consideration the insights and sensibilities of these faith communities when they legislate about "termination" of life, euthanasia, and the like.

Moderns cannot assent wholesale to the substance of all the religions around them; most of them contradict each other in many details, and some of them are in open conflict with each other—or divided within. Thus they present themselves as competing factions to scientists, ethicists, and legislators. Some observers may find them all to be fossilized, pesky, irrelevant, idiosyncratic, eccentric, partial, self-seeking interest groups. Yet others have come to recognize more positively much of what is in these heritages, or to value the efforts by contemporaries to come to terms with and to draw guidance from the traditions. These heritages make or may make positive contributions in mortal choices about times to be born and times to die and the ways of approaching both.

I am talking about an event that is occurring late in the twentieth century, an event that is Protean, whose components are diffuse, hard to discern and define, but that includes features that have manifest power. The notion of drawing guidance from ancient heritages in a postmodern world could not occur unless there were not some sort of opening in society, in the public order, and in the circles of those who must reason about mortal choices—including the patients, parents, citizens in general, who are often the most implicated people when it comes to making them.

The opening has a partly negative basis. The reassertive religions, however contradictory, conflictual, and—one must hypothesize or charge—"wrong" they may be, have caught the secular order in disarray. Vital in so many ways—technologically, politically, commercially— this order often lacks coherence or fails to address profound human needs in satisfying ways. Meanwhile critics of secular rationality within the philosophical community have contended and perhaps shown that the language of science and politics is, like that of the religions, somehow and in part "mythic."[14] This means that no single universal principle of reason moves the entire modern enterprise; that science operates within a set of changing paradigms that illustrate the partly mythic construct of each. Reason, argue not a few philosophers, is also conditioned by the persons who express it, colored by the communities that give expression to it. Faith communities, the Madisonians among 'us remind us, have as much right to speak up as do "reason" communities, as they often see themselves. Religion is not to be the element that disqualifies a person or community from seeking to make a contribution or to have her or its way in a republic.[15]

Mixed with this negative and defensive approach, which discerns a vacuum in the merely or utterly secular society, is a more positive set of understandings. In this set, it is credibly argued that there is no reason to restrict ethical discourse to people moved only by "secular rationality," a pattern that has come to make up the rules of the ethics game in modern republics. Most religions and religionists themselves today move by and are respectful of the modes of "secular rationality," but they do not want to grant it a monopoly in ethical inquiry.

Kent Greenawalt has suggested a better term than "secular rationality" as a basis for argument and inquiry. He proposes that, to be effective, the discourse must be "publicly accessible."[16] This means that a religious heritage cannot expect the larger society to be guided with what is hidden from other citizens who do not or cannot accept the content of a revelation that is not their own. James Madison never tired of reminding lawmakers that religion was at least a matter of opinion. Opinion could not be coerced, unless there were to be the creation of a republic of knaves, hypocrites, or fools.[17] Efforts by faith communities to impose policies based on their private revelations or formal dogma are rejected by a coalition that forms a majority against them or, where opposed by majorities, eventually come to be repealed. Thus rejection of anti-birth control statutes came when people perceived, rightly or wrongly, that legislation against artificial birth control was based on a revelation or a magisterial teaching that was not their own.[18]

While religious communities, therefore, have to use "reason" if they wish to make fair and effective argument, whether they appeal to "natural law" or "duty" or whatever else, they demonstrate to society that mortal choices made on other grounds are also publicly accessible. Religious heritages, though not they alone, move also by intuition, narrative, memory, symbol, community, affectivity, and tradition. Along the way they may, therefore, protect interests that cannot find a voice where secular rationality alone is at stake. Greenawalt illustrates this theme by showing religious interests in representing the natural environment, fetal, or animal rights.[19]

HOW TO: WHEN ADHERENTS DRAW ON HERITAGES

To this point I have discussed religious heritages in the plural and from the viewpoint of the larger society. But they come to the notice of society when living communities and their members speak up for these traditions. If legislators, ethicists, scientists, and physicians are to understand what they represent, our topic commits us also to inquiring how the representatives draw or can draw on the heritages. Hence the quaint and practical ring of the "how to" in our assignment. To the point: If there is an opening in the academy or the legislature, and if inheritors of traditions find voice to speak, how do they draw on the heritages? In the heritage of "how to" conventions, I will be enumerative and precise.

1. First, it is important to realize that there *are* heritages and that we are *in* them. Tribes may be aware that there are "others" in another valley, at the other end of their spears, accounted for in myths. But they may not realize that they are themselves "tribal," that the world they take for granted appears to all others to be an arcane and threatening or alluring but always different world view. Not to recognize this is to be a victim of inattentiveness, pluralistic ignorance, narcissism, or solipsism; it is to lack all perspective and distance.

"We" are in one or another tradition; in open and free societies characterized by much interaction of our "tribes" and reached by mass media of communication, most of us belong to many interactive, overlapping, sometimes fusing and syncretic, often apparently (at least in part) contradictory heritages. To be personal: I am a conscious heir of what often gets coded as Graeco-Roman traditions, through the classical tradition that undergirds the humanism behind the academy and the republic I cherish. Similarly, the heritage coded as Judaeo-Christian makes up much of the mental furnished apartment, the partly incommunicable world view I inhabit and choose to inhabit. Efforts by many brought up in such traditions to reject them often are so strenuous and demanding that they pay the traditions a compliment: It takes the energy of a whole life to "get out from under" what might be perceived as the repressive or dulling elements of such a tradition, but still one uses words or ideas from it as levers to turn it over and away.

Within these traditions, I am also moved by the Catholic heritage as transformed by the challenge of the Protestant Reformation. When I write on "health and medicine in the faith traditions," further, they assign me the task of articulating the Lutheran tradition, with which I am also critically at home.[20] But all these heritages get refined by the personal experiences and local adaptations.

No one pretends that these heritages are perfect matches for each other; they would not survive if they were. The "God" of the Republic—Nature's God, the God of Reason, of Law—was accessible, the Enlightened people of the eighteenth century believed, to all people of reason and good will.[21] This "God" does not match the "God" of revelation, who comes through a particular story about Israel and Jesus Christ and which has often been in contradiction to the civil faiths with which it coexists. Heirs of both find themselves dealing with what Alfred Schutz calls "multiple realities," and are, in William James's terms, "attentive" to more than one set of influences at the same time, even if these seem to be partly contradictory.[22] The heart has its reasons that reason does not know, but reason also has reasons. The main first point is simply to suggest that people have to be conscious that they are in a heritage, in heritages; that they do not have direct access to truth unconditioned by history; or that they cannot avoid being seen as deluded if they make the claim that they alone do not have a world view, an inherited framework.

2. To be "in" a heritage is not enough; if one is to draw guidance from it, there has to be some knowledge of what is in that heritage. Jaroslav Pelikan, writing in vindication of the Christian tradition, told about the time choreographer Jerome Robbins was asked to work with *Fiddler on the Roof*, which focused on a dying tradition. Robbins insisted that the important thing to know first was what the tradition *was*.

Such knowledge is difficult in the modern world. Most of us inherit traditions without being aware of them in conscious and articulate ways. They come as "package deals." Many of us are busy rejecting our own traditions. There is no reason for people to draw guidance only from the heritage that is theirs by the accident of birth. They can do philosophical shopping and slumming, make themselves open to conversion, go on intellectual searches, and they do. Religious heritages can represent death instead of birth and life. They can repress, stultify, and dull ethical response. They may offer substance, but the chalice is poisoned.

Further, there is widespread amnesia within the heritages. We ignore what we are ignorant of. The primary and even secondary associations of our society give the particular heritages little support. We live in a "pluralization of life-worlds." Nothing the Orthodox Jewish child confronts specifically as part of a religious heritage in home or synagogue will be confirmed in public school, over television, or among playmates in a diverse neighborhood. It is easy to forget as one goes through the passages of life.[23]

To the problems of unconsciousness, rejection, and amnesia one adds the fact that we often have grasped a heritage wrong. One inherits but never appropriates it with measurable accuracy. Many Catholics were surprised to hear what the teaching of their church was or could be when mortal choices came up in the famed Karen Quinlan case. There are often life-protecting or liberating elements in traditions that postadolescents overlook because in adolescence other and more deadening or repressive elements of the same tradition were imposed on them as if these exhausted the tradition. They rebel and distort.

This leads up to the understanding that one cannot draw guidance from a tradition of which one becomes conscious, respectful, aware, and that one gets "right," unless there is some knowledge of the content, substance, and detail of the heritage; one needs some cognitive grasp. It may not have been necessary to be so attentive to this when a tradition had a monopoly, as Catholicism did in the West for a millennium, or when everyone in your village lived by it. Jacob Burckhardt points out that we often do not write down the most important things in life simply because they are so obvious, so close. But in modern pluralism it is necessary to write things down, or to draw clues from what has been written down.

To illustrate: When I was to write on the Lutheran heritage, I put computers to work and probed many libraries. The specific tradition is 450 years old; 70,000,000 people call themselves Lutheran. Most sermons, classes, pastoral acts in the tradition assume that it has something to say about mortal choices, about being born and dying. Yet I could find no collection, no compendium, no systematic address to this urgent set of issues.[24] A dozen other authors in a series of books on the traditions report their astonishment at finding the same situation in their own.[25] In a world of choice, one must know what is available, what one has to offer or is getting. So in a secular, pluralist, liberal, scientific society it has become necessary and attractive to come to cognitive terms with heritages as one did not formerly need to do.

What, one might ask, does "knowing" a heritage mean? In the most forthright way, it implies taking some measure of possession. It is often observed that a convert does this best; she comes to a faith and is more alert than are those who merely inherited it. The living heritage satisfies a quest, beckons to deeper levels, and offers a repository of options that demand self-conscious appropriation. Not all members of the community do this taking of possession, but one expects professors, ethicists, clerics, counsellors, teachers, pastors, communicators, and leaders to have some awareness of what is there.

Where one does not take possession of a heritage, it is important to recognize that, as Eugene Goodheart puts it, a heritage possesses you.[26] This is the way most lay people who have no vocation to be self-conscious find the tradition. The words, gestures, expectations, behavior, symbols, and patterns belong to the reflexive world and one need not be fully conscious of them in order to draw on them. Not all Catholics have read papal encyclicals on the dignity of human life, but through the confessional, through public activities of their Church, they have absorbed the teaching, even if only partially and with some distortion.

3.   Drawing guidance from a heritage means trying to discern its core. As traditions move through history, they gain many accidental and apparently trivial elements. Yet they also have some root expressions and interests. The pope is reaching into something very near the heart of Catholic understandings of the image of God when he stresses "the dignity of human life" behind the ethics of choice. This is not the place to try to illustrate in detail; I shall only point. Somewhere along the way understandings of Jewish ethics in respect to being born and dying will deal with the notion of covenant. The physician, I have heard thinkers in this tradition say, will not enter into a covenant with a patient of a sort that leads the patient to fear that the physician will choose to be the agent of the patient's death. This may not be the only word such a Jewish physician has to say about passive euthanasia or termination, but it will color the relation.

In our series of inquiries we learned that within Protestantism, the Reformed (Calvinist/Zwinglian) heritage has a somewhat different view of suffering than does the Lutheran. There is more of a "taking command" under the sovereignty of God, more of an impulse to fight injustice and thus contribute to life, within Reformed Protestantism.[27] The Lutheran concept, while by no means passive or contributing to a cult of suffering, was more ready to approach it through the core teaching of grace and to ask for ministries of mercy, not justice. Islam has distinctive views of the limits Allah himself placed on life, and develops an ethic out of this.[28] The core of traditions is most obvious when we deal with those whose attitudes toward healing are easily recognizable: Christian Science, Seventh-Day Adventism, Pentecostalisms.

The teachings of these traditions do not appear as dogmas unconnected with each other. The reason it is hard to "move" magisterial Catholicism on the issue of abortion is that its position is grounded in a view of the transmission of life which is located near the center of what that church regards as "natural." The fundamentalist Protestant knows that in the public order she must similarly make a "natural" or otherwise publicly accessible case, but it is hard to "move" her because she sees this understanding confirmed in revelation, specifically through several biblical passages. Liberal Protestantisms may be as eager to protect life, but they may have other definitions of the status of life in respect to fetal or comatose existence; here theological doctrines of "rights" to which such Protestantism helped give birth or which influenced it are part of the core and have to be reckoned with.

The best "how to" advice, both for those in a tradition and those who would and must deal with it strategically, is to make an effort to find central and grounding themes, of which other teachings and ideas are corollaries.[29]

4. Although one may locate a focal or core theme about life and death in religious heritages, if one is to get guidance from them, it is important to recognize that one cannot get at such traditions *immediately.* They are mediated by a complex history. Something has happened to them. I recognize that what I am about to say will not be easily accepted by fundamentalists in the various heritages, though they treat all other fundamentalisms and heritages as I shall treat any one of them. This is a way of saying that a certain attitude toward history and interpretation is part of the nonnegotiable core of fundamentalisms, be they Jewish, Islamic, Catholic, or Protestant.

When dealing with one's own or another heritage, outside of fundamentalisms, one admittedly employs and understands hermeneutics.[30] By that I mean at this moment nothing more than the recognition that in dealing with either the parts or the whole of a textual or lived tradition, its partisans *bring* some assumptions, born of community and their own experience, and that these color what they *take* from it. Propose a basic text from the Hebrew Scriptures—say, the "suffering servant" passage from the Second Isaiah—and ask an informed, serious Jew, Christian, or Muslim to interpret it; and you will likely be able to anticipate some basic conflicts that will be forthcoming in the interpretations. This does not mean that there is no growth, never conversion, not any movement toward new understandings or convergences. It only means that the heritages come to us with a certain "thickness," and that drawing guidance from them implies reckoning with that density born of a community's experience.

The hermeneutic understanding is born of our passage into modernity, a world of plural understandings, of interpretation and criticism. In a familiar passage, Paul Ricoeur talks about what we might think of as a loss of innocence. It is impossible for us to live in the thought world of those who first received the revelation and transmitted it, who wrote the texts and lived off them. We may once have lived there with the "primary naivete" of the child, when first we were taught the myths, told the stories, or were given the doctrines. But then in the pluralist world that affects universities, legislators, and clinics, we pass into a sphere of interpretation and criticism. Now we have the choice to repudiate the tradition and its myth. Or we can continue to interpret "in spite of" interpretation—as the fundamentalist, often with some creativity, does. Or, still further, we can acquire a "second naivete" that appropriates the myth, the teaching, the doctrine, by leading one to believe not in spite of but *through* interpretation.[31]

Thus a Richard McCormick or David Ellenson can be believers in and adherents of a heritage and what it represents, and can be so with integrity. They can be even more informed about the detail of that tradition than many who have lived it in the past. But they are aware of other myths and world views, other heritages; they are alert to the meaning of symbols, allegory, or the complexity of the "literal" appropriation of a heritage. This means that the act of "drawing guidance" was more difficult when there was only one interpretive scheme per culture and a person could make decisions about birth and death without having a distance of any sort on one's heritage, or without being aware of others. This hermeneutical understanding, by the way, is what makes nonfundamentalist heritages somewhat more open to negotiation than fundamentalist ones.

5. Even with hermeneutical awareness, the politics of pluralism make the act of "being guided" complicated. A simple scene suggests this. A Seventh-Day Adventist is "brain dead." At the head of the bed is his pastor, who announces that the patient is ready for eternity; that nothing in the teaching of the Adventists, nothing in the family understanding, nothing in the expressed will of the patient, demands continuing life-support. At the foot of the bed is an Orthodox Jewish physician, whose Jewish concept of the physician's covenant and whose understanding of Hippocrates does not permit him to be an agent, however passively, of the patient's death. At the side of the bed (or down the corridor) is the staff ethicist, whose understandings are informed by Aristotle, Kant, Mill, and Rawls, and who must negotiate on the basis of "secular rationality" in an aspiration toward a universal language. All this occurs in a Catholic hospital, and its policies have to be taken into consideration. In the next room is another patient in similar circumstances, but other traditions are present.

It is not very therapeutic or cheering simply to have described how hard it is to draw on religious heritages, to be reminded of the realistic situation. I bring this up not to cause despair about the possibility of any communication but to suggest a framework for guidance. Although it is more difficult to find a path through the mazeways modernity creates, I would argue that the family and the society are better off for the necessity of drawing on various partly competing resources than would be the case if only one system were imposed "heteronomously," or if the culture were casual and moved hastily. One part of the "how to" theme in respect to heritages for guidance is the counsel to be patient, to listen, to enlarge the number of considerations before decision.

6.   Another way to draw for guidance on a heritage is to be open to communication and mutual influence among heritages. It is possible to *over*draw the picture of pluralism, to suggest nothing but chaos. Very often, perhaps almost always, mortal choices come down to two options, and a variety of philosophical and religious traditions bring different colorings to them. Philosophy has its sects, and the utilitarian, the consequentialist, the instrumentalist, the idealist, the pragmatist ethicist cannot each have his or her own way without reckoning with others. Similarly, in religion: These days some decisions made about nature and the environment and about human life in them are made by Westerners after they gain fresh insight from Native American and even Buddhist or Hindu views of time, mortality, and life.

The purpose of understanding traditions is not only so that one gets stuck or content with one, but with the possibility that one can learn from the conversation with strange, alien, "other" ones. The interaction enlivens each tradition and may deepen motivations for using as broad a repository of options as possible in each case.

7.   How do we draw guidance from a religious heritage? In our situation if the pluralist condition is taken into consideration, one must say: "carefully, critically." Pope John XXIII used to tell religious orders that they should reform in the light of the intentions of their founders, to whom they could not go back. Some literalists may contend otherwise— without convincing anyone but themselves—but most passionate adherents to religious faiths recognize that the same impulse that liberates may have a repressive side; that not all past teachings are available, to be imposed today. Some psychological understandings promoted guilt, which was death-dealing; contemporary articulators of the tradition need not be burdened by them. Inevitably, prescientific concepts led most ancient traditions to make commitments or applications that are irrelevant in the presence of new discoveries. Many heritages, for instance, changed their attitudes toward autopsy, cremation, birth control, and life-support, not by denying the tradition but by disinterring some previously overlooked meanings. "Stewardship of the earth," for instance, was a legitimate, available concept in their heritage that led mainstream Protestantism to accept birth control after generally having opposed it earlier. This change, for better or worse as others may regard it, was not done as an act of betrayal but of critical discernment and in order to propose new bases for choice.

To the cultured despiser of religion, the fundamentalist will often appear to be the believer with most integrity because of apparent intransigence. (I can show how fundamentalisms change, too, but that is not the present point.) Yet Catholic change does not lack integrity when it moves with its own concept of "the development of doctrine." Islam is not faithless when it accepts medical discoveries because the tradition says that "miracle" is worked through medicine, not by supernatural interventions.

8. How do we draw guidance from religious heritages? Increasingly an answer has to include the notion: by not claiming too much. For centuries, when religion was on the defensive in the West, its advocates, in sullen and resentful fashion, made apologias for religion in general. In the process they overadvertised the potential but ignored the contribution of particular traditions. Today, when there is the beginning of a renewed openness to the heritages, it is tempting once again to overadvertise the insights of religion. Although it is not my business to intrude on any particular faith tradition, it is not out of line as a historian or culture critic to observe that modest claims seem more in line with the heritages. Most of them do not offer fully satisfying theodicies or absolutist bases for having the right answers in ethical matters. The prophets and saints struggle, doubt, reverse themselves. They deal with paradox and ambiguity. New triumphalisms or religious imperialisms may be inevitable—one cannot easily talk a fanatic out of her fanaticism, the absolutist out of his absolutism—but the questioner can creatively complicate the conversation.

9. Part of the understanding of limits has to do with the location of religious faith. Its insights belong to the humanistic more than the scientific vision, though we must not overdraw the lines between these zones. I mean to say only that science looks forward; children may pass Euclid or Pythagoras in their knowledge about mathematics, and science keeps eating up its own past, abolishing much of what had been known as new discovery comes.

In the humanities, one more likely looks backward, to Mozart and Shakespeare, to Confucius and Maimonides, to Aquinas and Calvin and al-Ghazzali. The ethical thinker in religious traditions, perhaps more than the one moved only by "secular rationality," is likely to bewilder colleagues who address each birth-and-death decision on more purely scientific grounds. Why pay attention to what was said so long ago, before people knew what we now know?

The partisan of a religious heritage may be thoroughly at home with modernity, criticism, science, and technology. But she believes that the classics of the religious past were born of a sense of revelation, a manifestation of genius, an awareness of "epiphanies" that made the bearers particularly alert to eternal, transcendent, or sacral modes of being. We may not have that alertness or even much access to those modes of being, except through the texts and the heritages. But those who listen to the wisdom of the heritages, recognizing the depth of genius and insight, have a sense that, as I like to say by conflating two claims,

"They knew back there already what we do not know as yet." Patient listening to clues about life and death from times before there was genetic experiment, *in vitro* fertilization, or technological intensive care may serve to help contemporaries protect some values that the present-day economy, pace, and knowledge may obscure. One draws on a heritage for guidance by listening to those voices and listening for the clues. Thus the listener is not so much the rival as the complementer to other agents in the team of those who make ethical decision.

10. Finally, one recognizes that the heritages are vital not simply because they survive in inherited texts but are nurtured in living communities. They are not merely substantive ancient deposits, sets of doctrines, well-told stories and allegories. They surround living participants with meanings and gestures. They thrive as people become habituated to their ways. To illustrate: While writing on the Lutheran tradition, I asked a presiding bishop what advice he would give to a Lutheran who just learned she had a terminal disease. His answer: It would be good advice for her to have been an active participant in a lively congregation for twenty years.[32] There was wisdom of the tradition evident in that observation. Not that a convert cannot quickly discern meanings and acquire benefits. But much of the concern about birth and death, about time and choice, is nurtured in thousands of little decisions in the course of a way of life shared by fellow-believers.

The traditions may have much of intellectual bearing about them, but drawing guidance from them demands coming to know how and why people around us live by them. Only then can one gain the insight to recognize the power in the communities that embody these heritages. More likely then one is able to make judgments about which assertions of each heritage about mortal choice have to be taken seriously, for we can observe the motivations and the consequences in these living exemplifications of what would otherwise be heritages that lived, or died, only in libraries and textbooks. The renewed vitality of some of these traditions impresses and stuns many who thought we had all that behind us. The complexity of these heritages bewilders us in our busy lives, for we cannot be informed about them all, including often our own, if we are in one at all. But this complexity also signals options and possibilities that we may have long overlooked, and whose claim to offer guidance is not so easily to be denied in the future.

NOTES AND REFERENCES

1. Ancient Greek, Buddhist, and Hindu religions, for instance, are said to have cyclical views of time, opposed to Jewish, Islamic, and Christian linear views, and these differences have a bearing on "mortal choice."

2. I am using "heritage" and "tradition" interchangeably. On the concept of tradition, see Edward Shils, *Tradition* (Chicago: University of Chicago Press, 1981) and Jaroslav Pelikan, *The Vindication of Tradition* (New Haven: Yale University Press, 1984).

3. See Phillip E. Hammond, *The Sacred in a Secular Age* (Berkeley: University of California Press, 1985) and David Martin, *A General Theory of Secularization* (Oxford: Blackwell, 1978).

4. An excellent treatment of "equal separation of church and state," which correlates the notions of no establishment, no privilege, but also no disability, may be found in Paul J. Weber, "James Madison and Religious Equality," *The Review of Politics* 44, 2 (April 1982): 163–186.

5. Robert Booth Fowler, *Unconventional Partners: Religion and Liberal Culture in the United States* (Grand Rapids, Michigan: Eerdmans, 1989), 1–15.

6. Peter Berger, *The Heretical Imperative: Contemporary Possibilities of Religious Affirmation* (Garden City, NY: Anchor Books, 1979), 2–3, 11–17, 95ff., on choosing; 26–31 on heresy.

7. William James, *The Varieties of Religious Experience* (Cambridge, MA: Harvard University Press, 1985), 34. Religion is "the feelings, acts, and experiences of individual men in their solitude."

8. Harvey Cox, "Ernest Bloch and 'The Pull of the Future,' " in *New Theology: No. 5*, Martin E. Marty and Dean G. Peerman, eds. (New York: Macmillan, 1968), 191–203.

9. See Karl Rahner, "Revelation," in *Sacramentum Mundi: An Encyclopedia of Theology*, Vol. 5 (New York: Herder and Herder, 1969); H. Wheeler Robinson, *Inspiration and Revelation in the Old Testament* (Oxford: Clarendon Press, 1956); A. J. Arberry, *Revelation and Reason in Islam* (London: Allen and Unwin, 1957).

10. On exclusivism, see especially the work of Wilfred Cantwell Smith, including *The Meaning and End of Religion* (London: SPCK, 1978) and *Problems of Religious Pluralism* (London: SPCK, 1985); see also Harold G. Coward, *Pluralism: Challenge to World Religions* (New York: Orbis Books, 1985) and, for a Christian interpretation, Paul Knitter, *No Other Name? A Critical Survey of Christian Attitudes to World Religions* (New York: Orbis Books, 1985).

11. Charles Taylor, *Sources of the Self: The Making of the Modern Identity* (Cambridge, MA: Harvard University Press, 1989). See especially Chap. 15, "Conclusion: The Conflicts of Modernity," 495–521.

12. Taylor, *op. cit.*, is a book-length treatment of this issue and merits consideration for context here.

13. The political context for this medical and moral argument is Kent Greenawalt, *Religious Convictions and Political Choice* (New York: Oxford University Press, 1988), 21–25, 149–150.

14. See, as examples, Michael Polanyi, *Personal Knowledge* (London: Routledge and Kegan Paul, 1958); Thomas S. Kuhn, *The Structure of Scientific Revolutions* (Chicago: University of Chicago Press, 1962); Stephen Toulmin, *Human Understanding, The Collective Use and Evolution of Concepts* (Princeton: Princeton University Press, 1972).

15. See Greenawalt, *op. cit.*, 20–21, 34, 69–76, 112–113, 159–163, 208–211, 216–222.

16. *Ibid.*, 57–63, 70–71, 109.

17.   On the Madisonian approach, see Martin E. Marty, "The Virginia Statute Two Hundred Years Later," in *The Virginia Statute for Religious Freedom: Its Evolution and Consequences in American History*, Merrill D. Peterson and Robert C. Vaughan, eds. (New York: Cambridge University Press, 1988), 1–21.

18.   For comment on this issue and the problem of abortion, see Richard P. McBrien, *Caesar's Coin: Religion and Politics in America* (New York: Macmillan, 1987), 135–168.

19.   Greenawalt, *op. cit.*, 125–131, 147.

20.   Martin E. Marty, *Health and Medicine in the Lutheran Tradition* (New York: Crossroad Publishing Co., 1983).

21.   For an admittedly controversial but still appropriate argument on this theme, see Walter Berns, *The First Amendment and the Future of American Democracy* (New York: Basic Books, 1976), 1–32.

22.   See Helmut R. Wagner, *Alfred Schutz: An Intellectual Biography* (Chicago: University of Chicago Press, 1983), 90; William James, *The Principles of Psychology*, Vol. 1 (Cambridge, MA: Harvard University Press, 1981), 380–382, 386, 401.

23.   Peter Berger magisterially rings the changes on these themes in Peter Berger, Brigitte Berger, and Hansfried Kellner, *The Homeless Mind* (New York: Random House, 1973) and with Thomas Luckmann in *The Social Construction of Reality* (Garden City, NY: Doubleday, 1966).

24.   Marty, *Health and Medicine in the Lutheran Tradition*, 9.

25.   See the series of books on faith traditions published under the auspices of the Park Ridge Center, 676 N. St. Clair, Chicago, IL 60611. Volumes have appeared on the Hindu, Islamic, Jewish, Catholic, Reformed, Anglican, Methodist, and other heritages, while at least a dozen more books are being written.

26.   Eugene Goodheart, *Culture and the Radical Conscience* (Cambridge, MA: Harvard University Press, 1973), 15–16, 31.

27.   See Kenneth L. Vaux, *Health and Medicine in the Reformed Tradition: Promise, Providence, and Care* (New York: Crossroad Publishing Co., 1984) in contrast to the Marty volume on Lutheranism.

28.   See Fazlur Rahman, *Health and Medicine in the Islamic Tradition* (New York: Crossroad Publishing Co., 1987).

29.   For elaboration of this argument in one instance, see Martin Marty, *Health and Medicine in the Lutheran Tradition*, 13.

30.   See Michael Aermarth, *Wilhem Dilthey: The Critique of Historical Reason* (Chicago: University of Chicago Press, 1978); Zygmunt Bauman, *Hermeneutics and Social Science* (New York: Columbia University Press, 1978); Hans-Georg Gadamer, *Truth and Method* (New York: Seabury Press, 1975); Richard E. Palmer, *Hermeneutics: Interpretation Theory in Schleiermacher, Dilthey, Heidegger, and Gadamer* (Evanston, IL: Northwestern University Press, 1969).

31.   Paul Ricoeur, *The Symbolism of Evil* (New York: Harper & Row, 1967), 351–352.

32.   Marty, *Health and Medicine in the Lutheran Tradition*, 170.

Biographical Sketch of the Contributors

George J. Annas is the Utley Professor of Law, Medicine, and Health Law at Boston University's Schools of Medicine and Public Health. He is the author of *The Rights of Hospital Patients* and *Judging Medicine* and co-editor of *Genetics and the Law* (3 volumes).

Daniel Callahan is co-founder and Director of the Hastings Center. He is the author of *Abortion: Law, Choice, and Morality; The Tyranny of Survival: On a Science of Technological Limits;* and *Setting Limits: Medical Goals in an Aging Society.*

James F. Childress is the Kyle Professor of Religious Studies and Professor of Medical Education at the University of Virginia's Department of Religious Studies. He is the author of *Who Should Decide? Paternalism in Health Care* and *Priorities in Biomedical Ethics.*

David H. Ellenson is Professor of Jewish Religious Thought at Hebrew Union College-Jewish Institute of Religion in Los Angeles, California. He is the author of *Tradition in Transition: Orthodoxy, Halakhah and the Boundaries of Modern Jewish Identity* and *Continuity and Innovation: Rabbi Esriel Hildesheimer and the Creation of a Modern Orthodoxy.*

Ronald M. Green is the John Phillips Professor of Religion and Adjunct Professor of Community and Family Medicine at the Medical School at Dartmouth College. He is the author of *Religious Reason: The Rational and Moral Basis of Religious Belief* and *Religion and Moral Reason: A New Method for Comparative Study.*

Leon R. Kass is the Addie Clark Harding Professor, The College and the Committee on Social Thought, The University of Chicago. He is the author of *Toward a More Natural Science: Biology and Human Affairs.*

Barry S. Kogan is Professor of Jewish Philosophy at Hebrew Union College-Jewish Institute of Religion, Cincinnati, Ohio, and Director of The Starkoff Institute of Ethics and Contemporary Moral Problems. He is the author of *Averroes and the Metaphysics of Causation* and editor of *Spinoza: A Tercentenary Perspective.*

Carol Levine is the Executive Director of the Citizens Commission on AIDS for New York City and Northern New Jersey. She is the editor of *Taking Sides: Clashing Views on Controversial Bioethical Issues* and *Cases in Bioethics: Selections from the Hastings Center Report.*

Ruth Macklin is Professor of Bioethics at the Albert Einstein College of Medicine in New York City. She is the author of *Mortal Choices: Ethical Dilemmas in Modern Medicine; Man, Mind and Morality: The Ethics of Behavior Control;* and coeditor of *Moral Problems in Medicine.*

Martin E. Marty is the Fairfax M. Cone Distinguished Service Professor of the History of Modern Christianity at the University of Chicago Divinity School. He is recent past president and now Senior-Scholar-in-Residence at the Park Ridge Center for the Study of Health, Faith and Ethics. He is the author of *Modern American Religion (1893–1919): The Irony of It All; Religion and Republic: The American Circumstance;* and *Health and Medicine in the Lutheran Tradition.*

Richard A. McCormick, S.J., is the John A. O'Brien Professor of Christian Ethics at the University of Notre Dame. He is the author of *How Brave a New World: Dilemmas in Bioethics; Notes on Moral Theology: 1965–1980, Medicine in the Catholic Tradition,* and editor of *Doing Evil to Achieve Good.*

Fred Rosner, M.D., is Professor of Medicine at the School of Medicine of the State University of New York at Stony Brook and Director of the Department of Medicine at the Long Island Jewish Medical Center. He is the author of *Modern Medicine and Jewish Law; Medicine in the Bible and Talmud; Modern Medicine and Jewish Ethics* and co-editor of *Jewish Bioethics* and *Medical Ethics: Jewish Moral, Ethical and Religious Principles in Medical Practice.*

Frank D. Seydel, M. Div., is Assistant Professor of Obstetrics and Gynecology, Director of the Alpha-Feto-Protein Laboratory, and Associate Director of the Pastoral Care Needs in Genetics Program at Georgetown University. He is the editor of *Resources for Clergy in Human Genetics Problems: A Selected Bibliography.*

Robert M. Veatch is Professor of Medical Ethics at the Joseph and Rose Kennedy Institute of Ethics at Georgetown University. He is the author of *Case Studies in Medical Ethics; Death, Dying and the Biological Revolution; A Theory of Medical Ethics;* and *Value-Freedom in Science and Technology.*

Leroy Walters is Director of the Center for Bioethics at the Joseph and Rose Kennedy Institute of Ethics, Associate Professor of Philosophy, and Adjunct Professor of Obstetrics and Gynecology at the Medical School, Georgetown University. He is the author of the annual *Bibliography of Bioethics* and co-editor of *Contemporary Issues in Bioethics.*

Mark Washofsky is Associate Professor of Rabbinics at the Hebrew Union College-Jewish Institute of Religion in Cincinnati, Ohio. He is the author of "Abortion, Halacha, and Reform Judaism" and "AIDS and Ethical Responsibility: Some Halachic Considerations."

Index